The Care of Distressed and Disturbed People

DISTRESS: Extreme pain or suffering
DISTURBED: Agitated, confused and perplexed

Chambers Twentieth Century Dictionary

The Care of Distressed and Disturbed People

A Work-Book for Students of Nursing

P. N. WATKINS, R.M.N., D.N., R.N.T.

J. L. GOODCHILD, R.M.N., S.R.N., R.N.T.

Department of Nursing Studies,
Ipswich Health District.

WILLIAM HEINEMANN MEDICAL BOOKS LTD
LONDON

First published 1980

ISBN 0 433 34892 5

Photoset, printed and bound
in Great Britain by
REDWOOD BURN LIMITED
Trowbridge & Esher

Contents

Preface

Over the years in which we have been involved with the professional development of students of nursing we have been greatly impressed by two educational arguments. First the view that teaching methods should be more active and learner-centred, and secondly that teaching should be much less classroom-orientated; that we should try instead to exploit more fully and effectively the learning potential of the students clinical placements. This work-book reflects these views.

Perhaps because man is inherently lazy, or perhaps because many of us have been conditioned by previous educational experiences to 'sit back and be taught', work-books tend to be something of a 'turn-off'; for that reason we have approached this book on a 'give a little, get a little' principle. Nevertheless, it is still for the students who enjoy the challenge of investigation and discovery; who respond to an increased responsibility for their own learning. This book makes extensive use of work assignments and case-study material, much of which requires the student to focus on specific nursing problems and their solutions. We have made the text generous and informative for a work-book, but in no way does it undermine or negate the students' responsibility for completing the assigned work, using the recommended sources of information, and their own clinical experiences.

The book is intended to be adaptable and flexible enough to meet the needs of those pursuing nursing courses at different levels. Thus in referring to students, we mean the term to include all learners who are studying nursing. Although written primarily with psychiatric nurses in mind we have throughout been aware of the needs of the students pursuing a general nursing course. Most of the topics covered by this book are relevant to the experience of the general nurse who is increasingly having to cope with alcohol-dependent, aggressive and suicidal patients. Many of the assignments, case-studies and problem situations contained in this book are readily transferrable to the medical setting. We have purposely not set out to produce a comprehensive text on psychiatry. This has already been competently achieved by many authors. This book deals with the 'core' of psychiatric nursing, the therapeutic care of distressed and disturbed people. Each unit explores a different emotional or behavioural problem and sets out to develop sufficient knowledge and skills to successfully manage and to help resolve such problems. We have tried to give a practical account, uncluttered with technical terminology and unnecessary theory, of the common problems the nurse will encounter – such as suicidal behaviour, aggression, confusion and anxiety. We have tried to highlight and encapsulate what we regard as the essence of psychiatric nursing as distinct from, but not in isolation from, the roles of other professional workers.

The development of social psychiatry in the U.K. in recent years has provided a stimulus and a challenge to all those involved in mental health care. It has involved workers other than the psychiatrists in key 'front-line roles'. Professions such as social work and occupational therapy have been quick to develop their skills and extend their roles to meet this need; psychiatric nursing has not responded so promptly. Few training programmes adequately prepare nurses to participate fully in milieu therapy and there is understandably a notable lack of confidence within the profession, which has a somewhat myopic view of its own role potential and therapeutic worth. We are not advocating a drift towards the more systematic psychotherapeutic or counselling role based on the American model; what is important is that nurses should learn to be more aware of the therapeutic elements in their relationships and contacts with patients, and seek to develop and use these more effectively to facilitate the patient's return to mental health. These thoughts we have tried to capture within the text of this book.

We are indebted to Mrs Bronwen Scott whose secretarial support, and above all patience, has assisted us enormously in the preparation of this book.

Guide for Students

I listen I forget,
I see I remember,
I do I understand.
OLD CHINESE PROVERB

We believe that learning by discovery can be both enjoyable and an efficient way to learn. This work-book reflects this view and we hope that you will find it informative, stimulating and fun to use. We are aware that some of you will have the benefit of tutorial supervision, while others will need to use the book largely unaided; we have therefore written this guide with the unsupported student in mind.

Although a number of the work assignments in this book require review and feedback from tutorial staff in order to gain most from them, many assignments can be usefully completed as personal study projects using the suggested sources of information, and by drawing on your personal clinical experience. The units can be completed in any order but clearly those on the nurse–patient relationship and mental health form a backcloth against which the rest of the book is set; these should be worked through first.

Some of the units relate closely to specific areas of your clinical experience; you will find it helpful to work through the unit on the withdrawn patient before or during your placement on a rehabilitation ward, and the unit on the confused patient during your psychogeriatric allocation. But of course the behavioural and emotional problems discussed in this book can be encountered in such diverse settings as the community, a medical ward, occupational therapy, etc., and therefore work on these topics can be linked either to your lecture programme or to contact with such problems.

Those of you pursuing a course of general nurse training will almost certainly experience aggressive behaviour and parasuicide during your placement in the Accident and Emergency department. You will find it helpful therefore to read the unit on aggression, and sections on suicide and attention-seeking behaviour, at that point in your training. You will almost certainly have contact with patients suffering from anorexia nervosa and psychosomatic disorders during your medical nursing experience and work on the section dealing with those topics can be best pursued then. The other topics explored in the book, for example depression, can helpfully be linked with your allocation for special experience in psychiatry.

More senior students may find the book useful for revision purposes. The case-study material, assignment work and text provides a useful framework for systematically reviewing your understanding of certain topics. Working through selected units will help you identify and remedy gaps in your knowledge and experience.

At the end of each unit you will find a list of references and suggestions for further reading. We have purposely selected widely used texts, most of which you will find in your nursing library. Reference to these works will assist you in completing the assigned work. For easy re-referral you will find it helpful to head your notes with the assignment number and unit title. A self-evaluation test follows each unit. You should note that these are not intended to comprehensively assess your knowledge but will give you a general guide to your grasp of a topic and will help reinforce certain key points.

Guide for Tutors

The benefit to be gained from the successful use of this work-book will be increased by the participation of teaching staff. The work produced by students will clearly be of a higher value when supervised and validated by their personal tutors. We hope you will find the material contained within the book a useful source when planning work for specific areas of experience. We ourselves have found it valuable to prescribe assignments from the book for appropriate study block programmes and subsequent clinical placements.

Assignments from the various units could be used as a basis for work-sheet exercises or group discussion during a study block. Assignments could be completed and submitted for marking during the following clinical placement. We have used interblock tutor marked assignments as part of our process of continuous assessment, and also as a basis for ward-based tutorials and seminars. Interblock assignments focus on, and make use of, clinical problems the student is likely to see and encourage an imaginative, thoughtful patient-centred approach to care. In addition, students in our experience appreciate the continued contact with teaching staff and the link between 'classroom and ward' that is facilitated by assignment work of this nature. Block assignments lend themselves to a variety of teaching methods and can therefore be adapted to the needs of the students and the preferred method of the tutor. In this way assignments may be used as problem-solving exercises, as a basis for role-playing or as buzz group sessions.

There are two basic alternative approaches to the use of this book: either whole units may be prescribed as a programme of work, or extracts from a number of units may be used. As an example of the latter – to highlight the close relationship between confusion and depression in the elderly, appropriate extracts from the two relevant units may be prescribed. Cross-reference points have been noted in the text with this in mind.

Tutors working in the general field will clearly need to be more selective in their use of this book. Much of the material could be usefully incorporated into your students unit of special experience in psychiatry, but there are assignments that would seem more appropriate to other areas of training experience. We can see for example the relevance of assignments on confusion to a student during allocation to a geriatric ward or units. Similarly, work could be assigned on the psychosomatic aspects of medicine during allocation to a medical ward, and assignments on aggression perhaps during casualty experience.

AN EXAMPLE OF WORK ASSIGNED ON 'TUTOR/STUDENT PRESCRIPTION PAD'

Work Assignments for Psycho-geriatric Module				
Study Block	*Assignment* Unit 6 Ass. 8	*Assignment* Unit 6 Ass. 9	*Assignment* Unit 6 Ass. 10 and 11 (role play)	*Assignment* Unit 3 Ass. 13 (problem solving)
Inter Block	*Assignment* Unit 6 Ass. 20 To be submitted for marking and personal tutorial	*Assignment* Unit 6 Ass. 19	———	*Assignment* Unit 3 Ass. 2 and 3 To be completed by end of placement for group seminar

Private study periods would be set aside during study block for completion of work.

Unit 1

Mental Health

INTRODUCTION

It might seem usual in starting a book on the care of disturbed and distressed people to discuss first what mental illness is. A more realistic point to begin, however, is to discuss what it is not; for this is the state, or as near to it as possible, towards which health education and the care and treatment of the mentally ill are aimed.

It is not of course sufficient to say that mental health is merely the absence of mental illness. A person may not be diagnosed as having a circulatory disorder but nevertheless the performance of his heart may be poor due to lack of exercise. This analogy can be applied to the mind. A person may not suffer from an anxiety state but is so inhibited and withdrawn that the quality of his life is reduced. We believe therefore it is possible to talk about positive mental health just as one would talk about positive physical health. Mental health is relative to the cultural background of the individual: what might be considered normal, healthy behaviour for a tribesman from the New Guinea Highlands would not necessarily be considered normal in Slough.

The aims of this unit are to develop your appreciation of the concept of mental health and your understanding of the different processes that occur within and around the individual which may contribute to this. The unit concludes with a discussion of the contemporary concepts of mental health problems and their relevance to nursing care.

1. What do you consider to be the attributes of the mentally healthy person? Compare your comments with those of others in your set.

2. Compare your conclusions with the WHO definition of mental health. To be reasonably accurate your conclusions should encompass the following points:

Fulfilment of basic needs and potentials.
Successful coping with stress and frustration.
Realistic perception of oneself and the environment.
Establishing and maintaining inter-personal relationships.
Successfully adjusting to the cultural norms and expectations of society.
Vitality and productivity.
Self-regard and regard for others.

These criteria will now be considered and an attempt made to illustrate how mental illness may arise when the criteria are not met.

The concept of a person having a set of requirements that are essential to its well-being is not difficult to understand. This is a particularly so in the case of physical requirements or needs, such as food or water. The concept also includes psychological needs, although their existence and origins are a more contentious issue.

3. Define an instinct.

4. To what extent can human behaviour be said to be directed by instinct?

In modern psychology it is usual to talk about needs rather than instincts. Needs may be classified as being physical, psychological or social in nature and a useful, although not necessarily comprehensive list, is given bv Maslow in his *Hierarchy of Human Needs* (1954).

The needs that are low in the hierarchy must be at least partially satisfied before those that are of higher rank order become operative. When the lower rank needs are satisified then the needs higher up the pyramid become important factors motivating an individual's behaviour. Classification of human needs varies considerably from one source to another.

5. Decide whether you would include the following in any list of important human needs:

Spiritual needs
The need for sexual activity
The need for mental and physical stimulus
The need for independence.

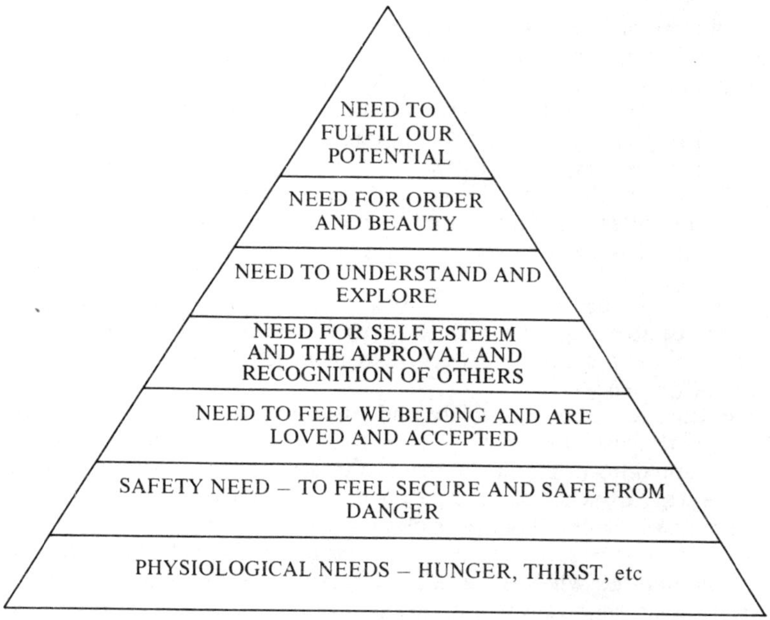

6. Consider how Maslow's *Hierarchy of Human Needs* may be used as a basis for assessing the nursing needs of patients.

It should be evident that it is possible for individuals not to fulfil all their needs, and that on occasions certain needs may be in conflict with one another. The conflict occurs when the fulfilment of one need results in another not being met. For example, striving for independence may well cause a feeling of insecurity. When needs are not being met, or are in conflict, the individual concerned may well experience a sense of frustration.

The way in which a person reacts to this frustration is very important. The temperament of a person is, at least to an extent, innate. Nevertheless the manner in which the persons react and cope whenever any of their needs are denied them, or are in conflict, is at least partially a learned response and begins from birth.

7. Consider how a five-year-old child may react when the needs at the base end of Maslow's pyramid are not met.

You can see that it would not be acceptable for an adult to react in some of these ways; although of course sometimes they do!

It is important for children to meet frustration, for this is how they learn to cope with it. For this reason it could be harmful to protect them from all frustrating situations. However, it is vital that the situation is within the resolving capacity of the child. One would expect a child to learn to resolve the frustrations felt when he had to chose between two desirable toys offered to him; one could hardly expect the same result if the choice was between two parents, as might occur in a broken marriage.

8. What might be the effect on a child who has over-indulgent parents?
You will be able to see that an adult's capacity to cope with stress cannot be measured along a standard norm, but is largely dependent on developmental experiences.

Children learn, both actively and passively, the differing methods of coping with frustration as they grow up. The mentally healthy adult will have adapted his behaviour to react to frustration in a socially accepted, mature way. Even so, under stress, a healthy adult may revert to methods more common in childhood, as a method of coping temporarily.

How does a person learn to adapt and adjust his behaviour in an acceptable manner when his needs are frustrated? The temperament has already been mentioned and this innate emotional tone provides the backcloth onto which experiences are built.

These experiences usually begin in the home and a child's parents are the first teachers. They actively teach the child limits of acceptable behaviour, codes of conduct and social expectations. They reward the desirable behaviour, and punish the undesirable. Just as important is the way they teach passively. The way they react to stress and frustration will be observed by the growing child and copied by him. In this sense parents are said to provide role models for the developing child.

Not only behaviour, but also attitudes and prejudices, may be transmitted in the same way. Obviously much of what a child learns in the early years will depend upon the conduct of the parents and on their limits of acceptability. The way they relate to each other and their environment provides a 'blueprint' for the child and may well influence later behaviour.

9. How might this learning be reinforced as the child grows older?
It is suggested by many authorities that the quality and nature of adult relationships is strongly influenced by inter-personal experiences occurring in the formative years.

10. Consider the immediate effects and long-term implications for mental health of the following examples of unfavourable early experience.

Parental rejection
Parental ambivalence
Parental overprotection.

Unhappy or unstable home backgrounds do not necessarily have a detrimental effect on the mental health of the children involved. Many persons suffering from mental illness had apparently happy, stable home backgrounds and many people who are mentally healthy personalities were exposed to very deprived circumstances. There are clearly other factors – such as constitution and subsequent experience – that influence the individual's development towards mental health.

Frustration results not only when basic needs are not fulfilled but also when a person has needs in conflict.

11. In what situations would the need for independence conflict with the need for safety and security? Comment on this in relation to adolescence, young adulthood and old age.

Although mental health is an individual state, it is, to an extent, determined by the accepted standards and beliefs held by the community. Such standards will vary from community to community and from culture to culture. What is considered healthy and normal in one culture may be considered unhealthy and abnormal in another. Thus to be considered healthy an individual must be able to recognise and conform to the norms of behaviour of the society in which he is living. To disregard these norms will inevitably result in punishment or rejection, and often both. It is possible that this is the main reason why people conform socially; however an internal moral censor is also an important influence on human behaviour.

12. Consider to what extent limits of behaviour are self-imposed by internal regulation and how much are they set externally by our society. Your investigation should include a consideration of the concept of conscience.

Prior to conformity the individual must first recognise and appreciate the relative importance of the society's norms. This is the first task of any immigrant when attempting to integrate into a new culture. In an attempt to conform they often mimic and exaggerate the customs of the society they have joined without fully understanding their value or importance. Thus in this country the situation arises in which some immigrants appear to be 'more English than the English'. Alternatively they may be forced to join their fellow countrymen in a sort of 'ghetto environment' in order to preserve the customs they understand.

13. Describe the problems faced by immigrant adolescents having to conform to a dual set of standards: that of their previous culture imposed by their parents and that of their new culture imposed by their peers.

Individuals leading reasonably gregarious lives will be faced frequently with situations that threaten their emotional equilibrium. These situations are unwelcome inasmuch as they hold the potential threat of insecurity and anxiety. Children face rivalry from brothers and sisters, students face examinations and the fear of failure. In a materialistic society many face the continual battle to maintain social status and all but the hermit face the fear of rejection and loss of valued relationships.

Apart from these general examples there are times in our lives when we are particularly vulnerable to stress. Such periods are the developmental milestones, for example starting work, getting married, retirement, etc., and are frequently associated with significant changes in the social role of the individual.

During the process of development we acquire and use a variety of manoeuvres which help protect us from emotional discomfort associated with stress situations and inner conflicts. These mental manoeuvres are called the mental defence mechanisms. They operate below the level of conscious awareness and we are therefore seldom aware of the influence they have on our behaviour. All mental mechanisms involve some degree of denial or distortion of reality or feelings, and therefore affect our capacity to behave in appropriate ways.

An appreciation of the nature of these mechanisms operating within ourselves and others will clearly help us become more rational and controlled in our behaviour and more understanding of the behaviour of others.

14. Make a list identifying situations that have occurred to you in the past few weeks in which you have felt frustrated or upset by people or events. Describe each situation briefly – they need not be particularly significant events; for example, the car wouldn't start, you burnt the toast, you had a row with a senior colleague, you got a poor grade in an exam. If you can't think of any examples this should be a lesson in itself!

Now go on to consider your reaction to each event and the way in which you coped with it; for example, got angry and threw the spanner at the cat. Can you identify any pattern in your handling of frustration?

15. The number of defence mechanisms vary according to the source but a generally accepted list is provided below. Find out about them.

repression	regression
displacement	projection
reaction–formation	denial
sublimation	dissociation
rationalisation	conversion
identification	introjection

16. Mental mechanisms may be both adaptive and maladaptive. Support this statement.

17. Suggest methods by which we might cope with stress in less defensive ways.

18. The following give you the opportunity to examine some situations and identify the mechanism operating in each case.

i. Ray is dropped from the local football team. He feels upset but says 'I don't really give a damn. I'll have more free time at the weekend now'.
Defence mechanism used:

ii. Terry is severely reprimanded by his father for a trivial matter and feels hard done by. Later his father finds all his tulips have been knocked down.
Defence mechanism used:

iii. Eight-year-old Janet seems pleased with the birth of her brother. However in the following weeks she begins to wet the bed and is very clinging.
Defence mechanism used:

iv. Ted's sales figures have been steadily dropping over the past few months because of his absenteeism. When challenged by his senior sales manager Ted angrily accuses him of being responsible by giving him the most difficult clients.
Defence mechanism used:

v. Unsure of how to cope with a difficult and demanding patient on

a busy medical ward, Jane uses the same brusque manner as the staff nurse when dealing with the patient.
Defence mechanism used:

vi. Although her parents are restrictive and overprotective in not allowing her to have boyfriends, Louise, who is an only child, does not feel angry and frustrated. In fact she seems to accept the situation unemotionally.
Defence mechanism used:

Finally the sense organs and the brain are the means by which the individual perceives the environment and their own relationship to it. Any impairment of the process of perception may potentially decrease the mental health of the individual. There are many factors both physical and psychological that can influence this process.

19. By considering the factors that might influence perception discuss the statement 'reality is in the eye of the beholder'.

20. How is perception altered in the illness schizophrenia?

All the topics we have been considering in this unit play their part in the formation and preservation of mental health.

21. What points would you consider important to include in a health education programme geared to improving the mental health of a community? Consider the application of the concepts of primary, secondary, and tertiary prevention to mental health problems.

THE MEDICAL MODEL

Historically this represents the first 'scientific' approach to mental illness. Physicians inherited responsibility for the care of the mentally ill by virtue of the fact that they were responsible for their physical welfare in the institutions and asylums in which they were kept.

Because of their training it was natural for physicians to regard the inmates' strange behaviour as being part of some physical disorder, and that the principles of management should be those used for physical disorder. As medical knowledge has progressed so the explanations of mental disorders in physical terms has become more research-based and persuasive. Abnormalities in the brain chemistry and genetic defects are currently offered as explanations for many of the common mental health problems. Physically based treatment has also developed over the years to become more sophisticated and selective. Malarial therapy and deep insulin therapy have been replaced by a vast armoury of psychotherapeutic drugs.

22. How might the illness schizophrenia be explained in medical model terms? What is likely to be the approach to treatment given this concept of the illness?

23. What effect might the medical model approach have on the patients' attitude towards their illness?

24. What type of role would be demanded of a nurse working in a treatment unit emphasising the medical model approach?

25. What are the advantages and disadvantages of the medical model approach?

THE SOCIAL MODEL

In this approach researchers stopped looking at the individual as a single functioning unit and looked instead at the 'ill' patient as being part of a wider problem. In this approach mental illness is regarded as arising as the result of a person no longer integrating in a healthy way within the social group to which he belongs. The family unit has been studied extensively since it is a microcosm of many larger social groups and the source of the most important and intense relationships which the individual experiences. It follows that if mental illness is seen as arising out of some group disharmony then the resolution is to be found within the disordered group and not through treating the individual in isolation. This has led to the growing trend for treatment to be community-based.

26. Outline the advantages and disadvantages of hospital-based treatment.

28. How might a treatment unit practising social psychiatry differ from one using a medical model approach? What are the implications, for the nurse and the patient, of this approach?

28. The disturbed behaviour of an individual can be seen as a symptom of a 'sick family'. Discuss this statement with reference to patients you have nursed, and comment on the implications for treatment of this concept.

THE PSYCHOLOGICAL MODEL

Much of the theoretical content for this model is the result of the work of the psychologist Sigmund Freud and other of his contemporaries. It basically concerns the study of the powerful, emotional forces which operate within and around the individual and which can undermine his mental equilibrium. According to this view conflicts and frustrations with strong emotional associations, often related to the events of childhood, can persist outside of our conscious awareness and have a considerable effect on our behaviour and emotional stability. As we have seen, the mental defence mechanisms are largely responsible for the unconscious nature of such conflicts and for the formation of symptoms in response to them.

29. How might a neurotic illness such as a conversion reaction be explained in terms of the psychological model?

30. What treatment techniques have evolved in association with this model of mental illness?

A more recent variant of the psychological model has been the behavioural model. In this approach deviant behaviour, for example excessive and inappropriate anxiety, is seen as being the result of conditioning experiences in early life. According to this view the individual may learn abnormal behaviour just as he learns normal healthy behaviour.

31. The behavioural model is largely based on the work of the psychologist B. F. Skinner and the physiologist I. Pavlov. Find out about their theories of operant and classical conditioning.

32. How might phobic anxiety be explained in terms of learning theory?

MENTAL HEALTH
Self-Evaluation Test

1. Neurosis can be basically interpreted as:
a. a maladaptive process;

b. a withdrawal from reality;
c. a process of intellectual deterioration;
d. a disintegration of personality.

2. In adolescence the term 'identity crisis' refers to:
a. a psychotic state characterised by memory loss;
b. a type of behaviour indicating homosexuality;
c. part of the process of achieving an adult personality;
d. the identity confusion experienced in early schizophrenia.

3. Statistics show that immigrants are a particular 'high-risk' group in the incidence of mental illness. This is because:
a. the National Health Service attracts many immigrants who are mentally ill;
b. mental health is better in integrated rather than disintegrated communities;
c. mental illness is hereditary in certain countries of origin;
d. many immigrants are mistakenly diagnosed as being mentally ill because of cultural differences.

4. Which of the following would be considered abnormal behaviour during adolescence?
a. inconsistent attitudes;
b. emotional equilibrium;
c. extreme anger;
d. intensive involvements?

5. Regression can be most accurately defined as:
a. banishment of unacceptable wishes or ideas from conscious awareness;
b. turning of interests inwards to total preoccupation with self;
c. unconscious efforts to eradicate a previous painful experience;
d. resumption of behaviour typical of an earlier level of development.

6. Denial can be best understood as:
a. keeping one trait unconscious by expression of contradictory behaviour;
b. unconscious refusal to recognise unwelcome thoughts and wishes;
c. an action designed to cover up unacceptable acts or wishes;
d. lying to others to cover up one's weaknesses.

7. Repression can be seen as:
- **a.** a process whereby emotionally painful conflicts and experiences are pushed into the unconscious;
- **b.** the process in which other's desirable attributes are incorporated into one's own personality;
- **c.** a form of self-denial aimed at relieving guilt;
- **d.** something that only occurs in neurotic illness.

8. Displacement serves the function of:
- **a.** disguising the user's personality weaknesses;
- **b.** explaining an individual's anti-social behaviour;
- **c.** allowing a person to study his own reponses to stress;
- **d.** providing an acceptable outlet for behaviour that might otherwise be unacceptable;

9. According to the most widely accepted theory, mental illness is most often caused by:
- **a.** a metabolic imbalance produced by dominant genetic influences;
- **b.** constitutionally weak personalities failing to mature properly;
- **c.** interaction of a variety of diverse social and biological factors;
- **d.** pressure from the sufferer's immediate social circle.

Assertion and reason

Each of the questions in this section consists of an assertion followed by a reason. Assign to each question one of the five categories (a – e) given in the key below:

KEY

- **a.** The assertion and reason are both true.
  The reason is a correct explanation of the assertion.
- **b.** The assertion and reason are both true.
  The reason is *not* a correct explanation of the assertion.
- **c.** The assertion is true but the reason is false.
- **d.** The assertion is false but the reason is true.
- **e.** The assertion and reason are both false.

ASSERTION

1. It is normal for a rational person to behave irrationally on occasions.

REASON

Individuals may be motivated by psychological forces of which they are not aware.

ASSERTION

2. Behaviour that is consistent with that demanded by a situation is usually regarded as being healthy.

REASON

Adaptability to differing situations is not a requirement of mental health.

ASSERTION

3. A degree of control over emotional expression has evolved in most social groups.

REASON

Overt emotional expression is good for the individual but bad for the group.

ASSERTION

4. It is usual to emotionally over-react when faced with increased pressure.

REASON

Individuals differ in the level of their general emotional reactions.

ASSERTION

5. The absence of abnormal behaviour in a sheltered supporting environment does not necessarily mean that an individual is mentally healthy.

REASON

Most behaviour can be seen as a result of the interplay between inner drives and environmental influences.

ASSERTION

6. Periods of frustration for the infant, if not excessive, are desirable during development.

REASON

Through experience of frustration children learn to modify and adapt their behaviour.

True/False items

1. There is a fixed criterion of mental health for any individual. (True; False)
2. Cultural 'norms' of behaviour should be considered when diagnosing mental illness. (True; False)
3. Greater preparation for developmental changes would probably reduce the incidence of some types of mental illness. (True; False)
4. Children should be protected from frustrating situations at all times. (True; False)
5. Most types of mental illness are inherited from parents. (True; False)
6. Constructive adaptation is a key feature of mental health. (True; False)
7. Psychological needs are less important as one grows older. (True; False)
8. The mechanism of identification is used extensively during the formative years. (True; False)
9. The use of mental defence mechanisms is valuable in maintaining psychological equilibrium. (True; False)
10. Personality development is likely to be impaired if parents project inconsistent attitudes toward their children. (True; False)

REFERENCES AND FURTHER READING

Holt, J. (1967), *How Children Learn*, Pitman Publishing Corp., USA and Penguin/Pelican, UK.

Hilgard, E., Atkinson, R. C. and Atkinson, R. L. (1975), *Introduction to Psychology*, 6th edition, Harcourt Brace Jovanovich.

James, D. E. (1970), *Introduction to Psychology*, Constable.

McCullough, J. W. and Prins, H. A. (1977), *Signs of Stress*, MacDonald & Evans.

Maslow, A. (1954), *Hierarchy of Human Needs*,

Mitchell, R. (1974). *Advances in Psychiatry*, Macmillan Journals Ltd.

Sainsbury, M. J. (1974), *Key to Psychiatry*, Harvey Miller & Medcalf.

Scheff, T. J. (ed.) (1967), *Mental Illness and Social Processes*, Harper & Row.

Valentine, C. W. (1956), *The Normal Child*, Penguin/Pelican.

Unit 2

The Nurse-Patient Relationship

INTRODUCTION

An important therapeutic influence to which a person is exposed on entering hospital is the experience of living in the social milieu of the hospital unit. Fundamental to this therapeutic experience are the relationships the person encounters, for it is largely through these relationships that his mental equilibrium is restored and he learns to live his life in more effective and fulfilling ways.

It is in this area of relationships that the main work of the psychiatric nurse lies. Through her interaction with patients she is able to provide comfort and encouragement, assistance with day-to-day living and help in resolving personal difficulties. Psychiatric nursing is of course no longer confined to institutional practice. The community nurse must make full and effective use of her relationship skills if she is to successfully support patients in their own homes.

The objective of this unit is to consider the nature of the nurse–patient relationship and to assist the nurse in forming and using such relationships beneficially.

Psychiatric nursing is often seen as taking the form of a multiplicity of roles.

1. Some of these role concepts are listed below. Describe the responsibilities of the nurse in these various roles.

- **i.** Technician
- **ii.** Social organiser
- **iii.** Teacher
- **iv.** Parent substitute
- **v.** Counsellor.

The emphasis which individual nurses give to the various role types in their work depends largely on the demands of the nursing situation, the needs and abilities of the nurse and, as we have seen in the last unit, the prevailing treatment ideology. Working in a psychogeriatric unit, for example, with very dependent and regressed patients perhaps lends itself best to the parent role. Patients are washed, bathed, dressed and fed in the caring and protective way we associate with mothering. There can be disadvantages however in giving too much emphasis to this role, particularly if the nurse has a need for patients to be dependent on her. In such situations she is unlikely to encourage independence by assisting patients to do what they can for themselves, and in so doing she will unwittingly contribute to the loss of personal dignity, morale and independence sadly so commonly experienced by elderly people resident in geriatric wards.

Some nurses, particularly those at an early stage in their careers, find informal interaction with patients stressful. This is perhaps because of a fear of rejection, or a fear of aggression, or because they are afraid they might say the wrong thing. They find it easier to function in a more detached technical role, and busy themselves with various tasks. By avoiding informal contact the nurse satisfies her own needs rather than the needs of her patients.

Other nurses involve themselves enthusiastically in social and occupational activities. Such activities are important in improving patients' social skill, confidence and self-esteem and in making their stay in hospital as pleasurable as possible. Not all nurses have the type of personality that lends itself to this role, and they function more effectively in one–one relationships with patients, listening to their worries and difficulties, providing support and encouragement and helping them to live their day-to-day lives more effectively.

Whichever role the nurse is adopting, her contact with patients will involve social interaction taking place, and it is the quality of this interaction that is of therapeutic significance.

Relationships arise out of social contact and interaction between two people, particularly when the contact has been a satisfying or rewarding one. Contact between the nurse and her patient should, if the nurse is able to recognise the patient's needs and to respond appropriately, lead to the development of a relationship that can be used in a therapeutically helpful way. The more contact the nurse has with her patient, and the more interaction that takes place between them, the more likely it becomes that a positive relationship will develop. Nurses need to be seen by their patients as available, approachable and helpful.

Although in psychiatry, and particularly in the therapeutic community setting, relationships between staff and patients become personalised, the nurse–patient relationship is different from a social relationship. Friendships always involve some degrees of mutuality – that is they are mutually rewarding – satisfying the social and psychological needs of the two people involved. In contrast the nurse– patient relationship is geared to the needs of the patient and not to the needs of the nurse.

2. Describe the ways in which those needs indicated below might prove unhelpful to the nurse in her relationship with patients.

i. Need for dominance
ii. Need for affection and approval
iii. Need for security.

Involvement is a much used and abused word. Effective psychiatric nursing by its very nature demands involvement with the patient in that genuine concern, warmth and interest must be shown. The term is more strictly applied, in the less desirable sense, to mean a relationship in which the nurse seeks to satisfy her own emotional needs and is thus unable to pursue her professional responsibilities objectively. Attitudes which sometimes indicate that a nurse has become over-involved with a patient are preoccupation with one specific patient, spending a disproportionate amount of time with that person, resenting other colleagues' approaches to that person, being unable to accept others' viewpoints, the expression of feelings of pity or anxiety or anger with regard to specific patients.

Nurses, like everyone else, have needs, feelings, attitudes and prejudices which will at some time or other get in the way of a helpful nurse–patient relationship. The therapeutic team should meet regularly to discuss such problems, for it is only through such objective discussion in a supporting atmosphere that we can gain insight into our own behaviour and 'grow' both personally and professionally.

3. What do you understand by the statement 'in a therapeutic community setting patients are sometimes staff and staff patients'.

4. You might find it helpful to complete the following attitude inventory. Discuss your responses with your set.

	Strongly Agree:	Strongly Disagree:
(1) Most mentally ill people are dangerous.		
(2) Most people who are mentally disturbed are overactive.		

Strongly Agree: | Strongly Disagree:

(3) People who have been diagnosed as mentally ill should not marry and have children.
(4) Alcoholics are people who are lacking in self-control and moral fibre.
(5) Proportionately the largest number of mentally ill people come from the lower social classes.
(6) People are usually admitted for psychiatric treatment in order to protect the community.
(7) Mental illness is like being pregnant: either you are or you are not mentally ill.
(8) Mentally ill people often have strong sexual urges which they are unable to control.
(9) People who are mentally ill should not be looked after in the community.
(10) Many people who are regarded as being mentally ill could 'snap out of it' if they really tried.
(11) Old people who are confused are best treated in a mental hospital.
(12) Individuals who persistently take overdoses are irresponsible and should be made to face the consequences of their behaviour.
(13) Mental illness and physical illness should not be treated in the same hospital.
(14) It is frequently necessary to isolate mentally ill people in a secure room.
(15) Mental problems are often caused by some disorder of the body.
(16) Mental patients should work harder to solve their problems, rather than waiting for the psychiatrists to cure them.
(17) There is really no such thing as mental illness; just people with problems.
(18) Mental hospitals should be abolished.
(19) Members of the medical and nursing pro-

	Strongly Agree:	Strongly Disagree:
fessions accept and have an understanding attitude towards mental illness, just as they have about other types of illness.		
(20) Anyone can suffer a mental illness.		

Many patients are people whose emotional or behavioural problems stem from their inability to establish and maintain social relationships. They are often lonely, isolated people who express their frustrations and despair in the form of anti-social behaviour, depression or self-injury. Often their need for attention and affection is so great that they may interpret the nurse's interest and concern as an expression of friendship in the social sense and may easily become dependent on her.

5. David D., aged 20, has been admitted to hospital a total of seven times, usually following some minor wrist-slashing or overdosing episode. Such episodes most often occur following family friction or some frustration or disappointment in his life. Nurse Jan C. spent quite a lot of time talking to David following his most recent admission and he appears more relaxed, confident and happy as the result of her interest. Now David seeks her out all the time, usually on some minor pretext. He tells Jan that she has helped him more than anybody else and that he can only talk to her. He has begun to ask her about her private life and is now asking to be allowed to visit her when he leaves hospital. Jan resents David monopolising her time, and does not want to further encourage his dependence on her, but she is also afraid he may injure himself again if she deliberately avoids him.

Discuss how this situation may be resolved.

6. A psychological process called transference may colour the relationship between staff and patients, particularly in situations where the nurse has worked closely with a particular patient.

Describe what is meant by the following terms:

i. Positive transference
ii. Negative transference.

Identification is a psychological process by which we model ourselves on the behaviour and attitudes of others, particularly those people we like and respect and whose approval we value. This process is important during early development for it is partly through identification with our parents, teachers and elders that we learn how to behave and acquire the standards, values and attitudes of our social group.

7. Miss Jill S., aged 18, who has been a patient in your unit for the past two weeks, was admitted following a threatened overdose over a bogus pregnancy. Jill must always be the centre of attention. She is noisy and flamboyant in her general behaviour and has a tendency to exaggerate the truth. Staff have noticed that if she feels in the slightest bit rejected or ignored she will quickly lose her temper. On other occasions she walks about the ward scantily dressed.

How could identification with a nurse be of benefit to this patient?

Identification may of course be a two-way process and a problem occasionally experienced by nurses early in their careers is that of over-identification with patients and their problems. While some degree of identification may help in allowing the nurse to respond in a more understanding and emphathic way, nurses sometimes feel quite intensely that they have the same, or similar, problems as their patients and this can arouse considerable anxiety. Although sometimes difficult it is important that nurses are able to leave their work behind when off duty and have absorbing interests and pastimes.

Mentally ill people need the opportunity to express and discuss their problems with someone who accepts them and has a genuine interest in their difficulties. The nurse in her counselling role deals with patients' 'here-and-now problems'. These may range from anxieties about coming into hospital, worries about how the family are coping, lack of progress, forthcoming treatment, other patients, not sleeping, and countless other things to problems of a deeper more personal nature such as relationship problems, financial or work stresses, sexual difficulties and feelings of inadequacy.

8. You are expecting the admission of Mr Jack C., aged 68, to the geriatric unit for investigation of confused behaviour. When you arrive at reception Mr C. and his wife are waiting. He is upset and angry about having to come into hospital, and his wife is obviously distressed by the situation.

Describe how you might help this man and his wife to accept hospitalisation and feel more at ease with the situation.

9. Mrs Janet F, aged 38, is a patient in your ward, suffering from depression. She confides that she hasn't been able to enjoy a normal sexual relationship with her husband just recently. She says she hasn't any interest in sex these days and is worried about her marriage and whether she is abnormal.
Describe how you might be able to reassure this patient.

An attitude of trust and acceptance are vital ingredients for the formation of a successful nurse–patient relationship. Trust in the staff will allow the patient to feel secure, confident and able to confide in them. It should be remembered that many patients, because of experiences of emotional rejection and deprivation in their early relationships, have become guarded, withdrawn and unhappy adults. Consistency and reliability in their approach to the patient by the nursing staff and an open friendly manner are important if a basis of trust is to be established.

10. Comment on the advantages and disadvantages of nurses wearing uniforms in psychiatric wards.

Acceptance is also an important element in such a relationship. This does not mean that a permissive attitude of 'anything goes' should prevail. Clearly, for the well-being of the patient and others, limits must be set. Acceptance means that the patient is not rejected or condemned for his deviant behaviour which is recognised as being an expression of his problems. Acceptance implies a belief in the basic worth of the individual and in his capacity to change.

11. Ian C., aged 20, has been a patient on your unit for two weeks and is depressed. Ian has been in conflict with people all his life and has never enjoyed secure lasting relationships with people, usually because of his anti-social behaviour or because of the excessive demands he makes of them. His mother died when he was 4 and he was brought up by his father, a strict and rather aloof man, and a housekeeper who was kind to Ian but was unable to express much emotional warmth. Ian was regarded as a trouble-maker at school and since his early teens has often been in trouble with the law. Since being in hospital he has been a model patient, but now the 'honeymoon' is over and he is refusing to attend the OT department, gets up late and regularly misses the morning meeting. At a staff meeting Nurse Jack C. says that Ian ought to be told to toe the line or get out.

Do you consider this the most helpful attitude or the best approach to the problem?

Relating to patients successfully involves the effective use of communication skills. Sensitivity to what is being said, either overtly or covertly, and the appropriateness of the nurse's response can significantly affect the development and helpfulness of the nurse–patient encounter. Communication between two or more people takes place both on non-verbal and verbal levels, some aspects of which will now be considered.

It is unlikely that patients will feel confident enough to confide in the nurse initially, and it is unwise to confront the patient with probing questions. During the 'getting to know you' phase, neutral topics of conversation best serve the purpose. Current local and national events, sport, hobbies and interests, the patient's job and family are usual topics to chat about. The nurse should be prepared to talk of her own ideas interests and opinions, but should avoid monopolising the conversation and answering questions of a private and personal nature. She should respond to questions such as: 'have you a boyfriend' by saying 'yes I have – but let's talk about you', indicating that the patient and his difficulties are her prime concern. Informal conversation, while primarily intended to build a relationship, can reveal a great deal about the patient's attitudes to himself and life, and often throws some light on his existing problems.

When a patient feels confident enough he will usually voluntarily discuss his difficulties. A more direct approach is, however, sometimes called for and the nurse must be sensitive to the individual's distress and the individual's need to unburden himself. The patient who appears unusually tense and withdrawn, for example, should be approached by the nurse who might say: 'you seem bothered by something this morning Mr C. Would it help to talk to me about it?'

Listening is an important facet of communication skill. The nurse, if she is going to engage in conversation with the patient, should sit beside him and inclined towards him. She should look at the patient, avoid fidgeting or gazing out of the window, nod her head from time to time and make comments such as 'yes', 'I see', 'go on', as appropriate. All of these things convey an attitude of attentiveness and interest and encourage patients to talk. If the nurse wishes to talk for any length of time and wishes to discuss some personal worry with him it is best to minimise distractions by talking in some quiet corner of the ward or suitable room.

The nurse should try and phrase her questions in such a way that the yes or no answers are inappropriate. 'Tell me about your weekend at home' is much better than 'did you have a good weekend at home?'

Nurses often find silences embarrassing and will immediately fill any lull in the conversation. This is not always desirable and the nurse should pause, remaining at ease and attentive, allowing the patient to reflect and collect his thoughts. It may be that he is building up the courage to say something important, and the tension generated by the silence may act as a spur. If the patient shows no sign of continuing he can be encouraged by referring to something he has previously spoken of – 'I was very interested in what you were saying about the demands of your job. Could you tell me a little more about that'. If this does not seem appropriate she should steer the conversation in some other direction by suggesting another topic. As her experience of interacting with patients increases, the nurse will find that many people have a tendency to trivialise conversation. This is best regarded as a defensive ploy which the patient adopts to protect himself from the emotional discomfort associated with discussing his personal difficulties. The nurse should gently point this out to the patient and provide sufficient reassurance and encouragement to allow the patient to be more forthcoming.

12. Discuss the nature and application of those 'reassurers' outlined below in nursing care:
Touch; Explanation; Proximity of the Nurse; Diversion and Displacement; Verbalisation and ventilation of fears and feelings; Counselling; Fulfilment of role expectations; Professional competence and composure; Familiarisation and the introduction of familiar elements into unfamiliar situations.

Some patients, because of the nature of their illness, have great difficulty in communicating with others. Such patients nevertheless find the companionship of the nurse comforting. Sitting quietly with the depressed or withdrawn patient, perhaps sharing a pot of tea or listening to a radio programme, can be greatly reassuring and may lead to effective communication later on. In her contact with withdrawn patients the nurse should be rewarding, in the behavioural sense, in response to any attempt by the patient at communication. Smiling and showing approval when a socially unresponsive patient says hello may reinforce this behaviour and increase the likelihood of his repeating it when the occasion again arises. Some nurses have a tendency to seek out and give most attention to patients who are socially responsive and relatively rational in their behaviour, and reduce the amount of time they spend with the aggressive, deluded or withdrawn patient with whom social contact may be stressful. Care must be taken to see that such patients do not become isolated, as they have the greatest need for interaction with the staff.

Patients may frequently ask for the advice and opinions of the nurse in order to help resolve their difficulties. While in some instances it may be appropriate to give advice, information, or to make suggestions, in general the nurse should avoid the temptation to offer pre-packaged solutions to people's problems. Patients should be encouraged, in their conversations with the nurse, to explore their difficulties so that they can come to see them more clearly and realistically. In time they will gain the insight and understanding necessary to arrive at their own solutions. In such situations the nurse acts as a mirror reflecting back to the patient a more objective picture of himself and his situation. Many patients with whom the nurse will have contact have a very confused and distorted view of themselves and the real world. In her conversations with such patients the nurse helps them test and retain contact with reality, and therefore to respond to their environment in a more rational and controlled way.

The ventilation of feelings and difficulties is in itself therapeutic. It releases tensions and generates the sense of relief that comes with sharing a problem. The nurse should remember, however, that it is often very difficult for people to express themselves freely in this way. They may later reprove themselves or feel guilty or embarrassed for having unburdened themselves to the nurse. It is important that the nurse does not convey disapproval or surprise, or become upset by what the patient may say or do. She should indicate that she is glad the patient has confided in her and that she can see how the situation must have been very difficult for him.

Having confided in the nurse the patient may request that she does not discuss what he has told her with anyone. The nurse should point out early in the conversation, if she anticipates such a request, that she must pass such information on to the charge-nurse and doctor, as they are part of the team engaged in helping the patient.

13. It is our view that much of the contact between patients and staff has a tendency to become inconsistent and ritualised. Often it has no clear objective and is of little therapeutic value. We suggest therefore, that from a training and therapeutic viewpoint, regular nurse–patient encounters with clear objectives supervised by clinical or tutorial staff would be of value.

We suggest the assignment outlined below may be carried out by the learner in different clinical placements throughout the training programme. It will be seen that assignments are geared towards improving relationships skills and achieving a therapeutic target. A progress record should be kept of each nurse–patient encounter by the learner and these should be evaluated at frequent intervals by supervising staff.

NURSE–PATIENT RELATIONSHIP PROCESS CHART

Clinical synopsis:

Objectives

For example, to build up confidence and self-esteem; to reduce tension, suspiciousness, guardedness; to reduce withdrawal, encourage spontaneity and assertiveness.

Initial contact

Here the nurse should record concisely her first contact with the patient; how she approached the task of 'breaking the ice' and facilitated the development of a relationship.

Record of Nurse–Patient meetings

Here the nurse should record a synopsis of each significant contact with the patient. She should comment concisely on the patient's responses, behaviour and feelings and on her own feelings and responses.

Evaluation with Supervisor:

Every social encounter relies a great deal on the effective use of body language. It is worth remembering that animals communicate almost entirely by this means, and it should therefore not be surprising that, despite a highly evolved and sophisticated language, we still make extensive use of non-verbal behaviour when communicating with each other. Social behaviour, such as smiling, eye contact, body postures, head nodding, hand gestures and variations in tone of voice signal our attentiveness to what is being said, communicates our attitudes and feelings and sometimes replaces speech altogether.

Body language is therefore of great significance to the nurse in her care of patients. Attitudes and feelings which have hindered social adjustment such as insecurity, self-centredness, excessive anxiety or aggression may be observed in the person's non-verbal behaviour. Anti-social or deviant acts such as window-smashing or wrist-cutting are clearly potent non-verbal expressions of unhappiness and frustration. Many of our patients experience great difficulty in communicating successfully with people and either because of, or as a prelude to illness, become increasingly isolated and deprived of the warm fulfilling experience of close human relationships. Often it is not so much verbal skill which is lacking but an adequate repertoire of body language. Such people can be helped by the use of group therapy and by role play, both of which may concentrate on developing social skills. Other patients who feel vulnerable and threatened by social encounters may use body language to discourage social contact. They may turn away when approached, look down at their feet, maintain a blank expression, adopt bizarre postures and mannerisms and, if they speak at all, speak inaudibly or incoherently.

14. Select a patient on your unit. Observe the non-verbal behaviour of this patient during personal contact with her and unobtrusively in different situations.
Tabulate your observations below:

Non-Verbal Behaviour:	*Reasons for Behaviour:*
(Example) Rapid foot-tapping throughout the conversation	Anxiety/tension experienced during social encounters.

Remember that it is not only the patient who is communicating in this way. The nurse also conveys her attitudes and feelings towards the patient, in her expressions, gestures and by the tone of her voice. Relationships sometimes fail to develop because, although the nurse may verbally convey an attitude of interest and concern, her expressions may be conveying dislike and disapproval. Conversely the nurse who appears rather gruff and authoritative in her approach to patients may be very successful in her relationships because non-verbally she conveys an attitude of kindness and concern.

Many authorities believe that it is best to avoid this incongruence between verbal and non-verbal behaviour and that an open and honest expression of attitudes and feelings in an atmosphere of acceptance is more likely to have a corrective and normalising influence on patients behaviour.

15. Discuss the advantages and disadvantages of this approach.

THE NURSE–PATIENT RELATIONSHIP

Self-Evaluation Test

1. An accepting attitude is an important prerequisite for the development of a helpful relationship. Acceptance means —. Select the best explanation from the list below:
a. the patient should be allowed to behave much as he likes while in hospital;
b. the nurse should accept the fact that the patient cannot help the way he behaves;
c. deviant behaviour should always be seen as an expression of the patient's problems and a belief in his basic worth should be maintained;
d. the nurse should regard deviant behaviour as a reflection of moral weakness.

2. A patient persistently seeks you out, often on minor problems, and is beginning to monopolise your time. Select from the list below the best solution to this problem:
a. tell him you are too busy to talk to him and hope he will eventually stop monopolising you;
b. encourage greater involvement with others;
c. try and keep out of his way;
d. always try and give him what time you can.

3. A colleague stops you in the corridor and tells you to stop involving yourself with a certain patient; she feels *she* is helping him. This is an example of:
a. transference;
b. identification;
c. over-involvement;
d. rationalisation.

4. Reassurance is an important element in patient care. Select from the list below those items which have a reassurance value:
a. being understood and listened to;
b. nurses who appear confident and competent;
c. becoming aware that others share similar problems;
d. clean, tidy, well-organised ward;

e. physical contact;
f. having things clearly explained.
(i) a,b,e,f
(ii) a,b,c,e
(iii) b,c,d,e
(iv) all of the above.

5. During a conversation with a patient you notice that he continually fidgets with his tie and taps his foot. This is *most* likely to be because of:
a. habit;
b. boredom;
c. emotional tension;
d. drug side-effect.

6. You notice Mrs G anxiously pacing the corridor of the ward. Select the best reponse from the list below:

a. let's go and find Sister, Mrs G., and see if you can have some tablets to help you relax;
b. go and sit in the day room and try and relax;
c. you seem bothered by something, Mrs G., would it help to talk to me about it?
d. it can't be all that bad, Mrs G., come and help me make the beds.

Assertion and reason

Each of the questions in this section consist of an assertion followed by a reason. Assign to each question one of the five categories (a–e) given in the key below.

KEY
a. The assertion and reason are both true.
The reason is a correct explanation of the assertion.
b. The assertion and reason are both true.
The reason is *not* a correct explanation of the assertion.
c. The assertion is true but the reason is false.
d. The assertion is false but the reason is true.
e. The assertion and reason are both false.

ASSERTION
1. Too much emphasis on the role of parent substitute may foster dependent behaviour in patients.

REASON
The nurse is fulfilling her own needs in this role and is not able to encourage self-reliance.

ASSERTION
2. The nurse–patient relationship is essentially no different from an ordinary social relationship.

REASON
In the nurse–patient encounters, the needs of the patient are the focus of the relationship.

ASSERTION
3. In the 'getting to know you' phase of a nurse–patient relationship, the nurse should be prepared to talk about her own ideas, interests and opinions.

REASON
A degree of familiarity is a necessary prerequisite for the development of any relationship.

ASSERTION
4. The nurse should promptly fill any silences during her conversations with patients.

REASON
Silences may act as the spur the patient needs to say something important.

ASSERTION
5. The nurse should never reveal her true feelings and opinions about a patient directly to the person concerned.

REASON
Psychiatric patients are emotionally fragile.

ASSERTION
6. It is most important that nurses do not convey disapproval or surprise at what patients confide in them.

REASON
The person may later feel self-reproachful, embarrassed or guilty for having unburdened himself.

ASSERTION
7. Patients will sometimes persistently focus conversation on trivial, inconsequential matters.

REASON
The patient regards a discussion of personal problems as outside the province of the nurse.

ASSERTION
8. The nurse's need for affection and approval may sometimes unhelpfully influence her approach to patient care.

REASON
She is unable to be objective and her actions are influenced by what the patient will approve of, rather than what the needs of the patient are.

True/False items

1. Imagining that you are 'losing your mind' may arise as the result of over-identification with patients. (True; False)
2. Nurses may seek to satisfy their need for dominance and authority by clinging to their uniforms. (True; False)
3. Assisting with E C T is an example of the technical role of the nurse. (True; False)
4. In most cases it is best to discharge unco-operative patients. (True; False)
5. Nurses should not become involved with their patients. (True; False)
6. In her counselling role, the nurse should confine herself to patients' 'here-and-now problems'. (True; False)

REFERENCES AND FURTHER READING

Altschull, A. (1972), *Patient–Nurse Interaction*, Churchill Livingstone.
—— (1978), *Psychiatric Nursing*, Baillière Tindall.
Argyle, M. (1972), *Psychology of Interpersonal Behaviour*, Pelican.

Cormack, D. (1976), *Psychiatric Nursing Observed*, R.C.N. Publications.
French, H. (1979), Reassurance: A nursing skill? *Journal of Advanced Nursing* vol. 4, No. 6.
Gillis, L. (1972), *Human Behaviour in Illness*, Faber.
Mereness, D. (1978), *Essentials of Psychiatric Nursing*, Mosby.
Towell, D. (1975), *Understanding Psychiatric Nursing*, R.C.N. Publications.

Unit 3

Nursing the Depressed Patient

INTRODUCTION

The therapeutic care and comfort of seriously depressed people, both at home and in hospital, is a common psychiatric nursing situation. Depression in its clinical form differs from the common experience of being 'fed up' or 'low in spirits' in that it is a more profound and enduring state that has a disruptive effect on the individual's life. It can range in severity from a feeling of fatigue, dejection and gloomy pessimism to states of depressive stupor in which the individual's mental and physical responsiveness is seriously retarded. Depression is also an illness that carries a relatively high mortality rate. Four thousand people kill themselves annually in the U.K. and it is estimated that at least one-third are suffering from depressive illness at the time of their suicide. Because of this close relationship we have included a discussion of the care of suicidal patients in this unit, although such behaviour is not exclusive to the depressive disorders.

The aim of this unit is to increase your understanding of depression and to help you develop a therapeutically helpful approach to patient care.

The diagram below represents a spectrum of human mood experience. For most of us the pendulum fluctuates back and forwards across the normal segment in response to the physiological rhythms of our bodies and our day-to-day experiences of frustration, pleasure and disappointment.

1. Try and recollect a recent personal experience of being 'depressed'. Briefly describe your feelings, behaviour and attitudes towards others.

Many quite profound and incapacitating mood experiences are also

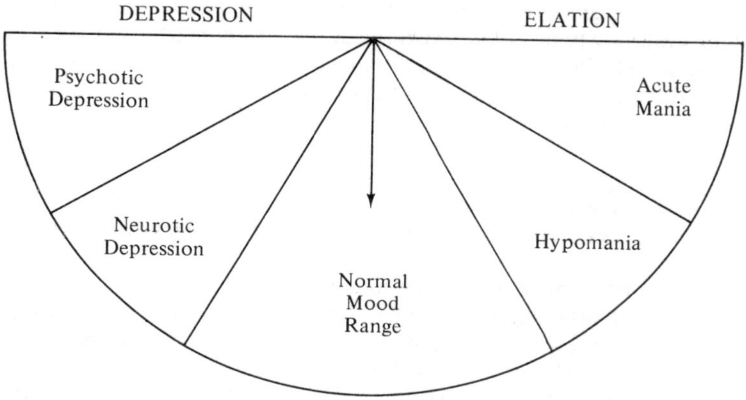

contained within this normal segment. They do not usually constitute depression in the clinical sense in that they are understandable and appropriate reactions to some stress experience and are usually transient, responding to the emotional support of family and friends. Some authorities regard depressive reactions of this type as being a feature of the minds of self-healing processes. It would appear that by lowering our general level of responsiveness we can make the necessary psychological adjustments to changing circumstances. The grief reaction is best seen as an example of this process. Rather than treatment in the formal sense, people need to be allowed to work through this experience in a comforting, supportive atmosphere.

2. In facing the crisis of loss, bereaved people are said to pass through various stages of grief (Parkes, 1972). Describe the behaviour characteristic of those stages listed below:

i. Anxiety and panic
ii. Denial and searching
iii. Anger and guilt
iv. Identification and mitigation.

It is clearly important that people are able to work through their grief and adjust to their loss. Sometimes people fail to do this and become 'fixated' at one or more of the above stages, thus allowing their grief to blight their personality and restrict their life. Those who may be vulnerable to an incapacitating grief reaction are isolated people, people who had a difficult or unhappy relationship with the deceased; those who had a very close, dependent relationship with the deceased and those who keep their feelings under strict control put on a brave face and need to maintain a posture of self-reliance.

3. Discuss the ways in which, as a professional helper or as a friend, you could help a bereaved person work through the stages described above.

Some authorities have noted a similarity between the grief reaction and the reaction to other significant loss, for example divorce, or amputation. Comment on this, referring if possible to patients you have nursed.

It has long been the practice to describe two diagnostic types of depressive illness – the neurotic (reactive) type and the more severe and incapacitating psychotic (endogenous) type. To some extent this is a misleading and arbitrary categorisation as environmental stress-precipitants are common to both types, and many depressions present with features normally ascribed to both.

4. Compare and contrast the main clinical features of these two types of depression.

Neurotic Depression	*Psychotic Depression*

The term unipolar depression is sometimes used to describe endogenous depression that is not associated with pathological mood swings towards the opposite pole of the mood spectrum. A disorder characterised by these extreme fluctuations in mood is called bipolar depression (manic-depressive psychosis) and is discussed later in the unit.

Many factors appear to interact to produce depressive illness. There is much evidence that certain individuals are predisposed genetically to suffer from depression. It is thought that this 'depressive gene' operates by producing a disturbance in the brain chemistry at the neuronal synaptic junctions. Recent research has also highlighted a relationship between a disturbance in body electrolytes and depression.

Some authorities emphasise the importance of changes in the blood hormone levels in emotional disturbance; certainly many women experience feelings of anxiety, depression, irritability and tiredness in addition to various physical symptoms, regularly, before the onset of menstruation. In a number of cases serious behavioural disturbance, for example suicide attempts or baby-battering, may be attributed to the 'pre-menstrual syndrome'.

5. Identify the ways in which your own mood and behaviour are influenced by your menstrual cycle.

6. Try and identify regular fluctuations in the mood, behaviour and physical symptoms of your patients that may be related to their menstrual cycle.

Others may be predisposed psychologically to suffer from depression. Some authorities suggest unresolved emotional conflicts associated with parental loss, or separation in early childhood, may be reactivated by stress situations involving the loss of someone or something significant to the individual in later life. An interesting view of depressive disorders of this type is that it arises as the result of distortions of the bonding process in childhood. Parker (1978) describes the key distortions as underbonding and overbonding. An underbonded relationship occurs as the result of maternal apathy, indifference or rejection. The consequence of this type of relationship may be that the development of the individual's self-esteem is stunted. He acquires a depressive disposition, adopting a gloomy, pessimistic, self-reproachful attitude to life and is over-sensitive to any hint of rejection or failure. Other individuals who have experienced underbonding seem on the whole to have better-adjusted personalities but are sensitised by key events in childhood, such as separation from parents, to situations in later life that 'mimic' the early event. In an overbonded relationship, perhaps because of mother's own emotional needs, the child is not encouraged towards independence and autonomy. The result is that such individuals are very dependent in their relationships and their self-esteem is externally regulated to an excessive degree. They seek always to please, to do the right thing, and are very sensitive to criticism and very vulnerable to distancing or rejection in their relationships.

A recent approach to the understanding of depression has come from the behaviourists. According to their view depression occurs when the individual comes to believe that his actions will make no difference to bringing about a change in a stressful situation. This phenomenon they term 'learnt-helplessness' (that is, a depressive reaction). A person faced in his formative years with stress situations which are beyond his resolving capacity may learn this maladaptive response and react in this way to difficulties with which he is confronted in later life, even though a solution may be within his capabilities. Support for this theory comes from experimental work with dogs. Animals exposed to stress situations from which there was no escape soon became passive, disinterested and helpless and later would remain so even when escape was perfectly possible. It required many trials in which the animals were made to take the avenue of escape before a new adaptive response occurred spontaneously.

7. What are the implications, for the management and treatment of depressed patients, of this theory?

These predisposing factors make the individual vulnerable to the many physical, social and psychological stresses to which we are exposed in our day-to-day lives. For a resumé of contemporary social stresses you may find it helpful to refer to Unit 4: 'Nursing the Anxious Patient'.

Although depression may occur at any age, including childhood, it is most common during certain developmental periods of life. Adolescence, marriage, parenthood, middle age and old age are important epochs in development which require psychological adjustments to be made in the changing social circumstances and physical capacities of the individual. These transition periods in our lives are often accompanied by considerable stress.

8. Describe the psychological and social difficulties with which the following individuals may be faced.

i. An 18-year-old male student in his first year at college
ii. A young mother with a new baby, living on a housing estate some distance from her parents
iii. A woman of 45 years of age whose family are growing up and leaving home
iv. A 65-year-old retired railwayman who has recently had a mild heart attack.

9. Depression is often associated with feelings of worthlessness, hopelessness and guilt. How could your approach to the care of the patient below help her regain a sense of personal esteem and encourage a feeling of optimism.

Mrs G., aged 52, has been depressed for five months. Recently her depression has become more incapacitating and she has been admitted to your unit for treatment. Mrs G. feels her family would be a lot better off without her and blames herself unreasonably for not being a better mother to her children and wife to her husband. She says she ought to be locked away and does not deserve the attention of anyone.

Guilt feelings often feature very prominently in depressive illness; many patients act and feel as if they have or are about to commit some crime.

10. What is the origin of such feelings?

Hypochondriacal ideas, sometimes taking a bizarre form, are quite common in depressive illness. This morbid preoccupation with body function and imaginary illness results from a misinterpretation of the physical sensation and symptoms experienced by anxious and depressed patients. The altered autonomic nervous system activity that occurs in these emotional states is responsible for many of these symptoms and sensations, e.g. constipation, dyspepsia.

11. How would you reassure a depressed and anxious patient who persistently complains that his 'insides are rotting away'.

The 'ventilation' of problems and emotions may be helpful to the depressed person and should be gently encouraged. The psychiatric nurse is in a somewhat unique position here in that, particularly during the early stages of hospitalisation, she is the member of the treatment team likely to have most contact with the patient during a period of high dependency. It is, therefore, likely that a relationship in which the patient feels confident enough to express his difficulties and feelings will occur.

The nurse must always be prepared to listen attentively and respond in an understanding way. Within the social milieu of the admission unit this outlet may also be provided by a fellow patient or a therapeutic group. It is important to appreciate, however, that in exposing themselves emotionally they may reinforce a view of themselves as being inadequate, and in doing so exacerbate feelings of hopelessness and despair. Understanding, coupled with the realisation that others share similar problems, can be a great source of support and comfort.

Forcing the depressed person to 'join in' and 'cheer up' is an unhelpful approach as it may increase feelings of self-deprecation. However, encouragement towards greater participation in suitable occupational and recreational activities can help towards recovery.

12. Select a patient on your ward and briefly describe his occupational programme, indicating how this can/has help(ed) the patient.

13. Neglect of personal appearance and hygiene, loss of appetite and weight, loss of libido, dyspepsia, constipation and headache are some of the physical features commonly associated with depression. Skilled nursing care is therefore required to prevent a deterioration in general health.

> **i.** List some of the reasons why a depressed patient may refuse meals
> **ii.** Suggest ways in which these problems you mention may be overcome.

14. Fatigue and insomnia are troublesome and distressing features of depression. Adequate rest and relaxation are therefore important factors in recovery.

Mr David F. was admitted to your unit two days ago in a seriously depressed state. It is now 4 a.m. and despite repeat sedation he is awake and restless. Why would you be particularly concerned about Mr F. and how would you deal with this problem?

15. In many cases of depression where the risk of suicide is considered minimal and intensive physical treatment is not indicated, treatment in the community may be the most desirable course of action. Say why this may be so.

16. John C., aged 32, has been depressed for three months. The onset apparently coincided with talk of redundancy at the factory where John is employed, and followed a bout of influenza. His GP is rather concerned as John is becoming increasingly tearful, morbidly preoccupied and is now unable to work. John's behaviour has also added a strain to an already unstable relationship with his wife. She feels John is rather spineless and has no 'go' or ambition. She complains that he tends to leave all the important family decisions and responsibilities to her, and that their life has not matched the expectations she held when they got married. John's GP has now referred him to the community psychiatric team.

As a member of the community team assigned to visit John, discuss what you consider to be the most helpful way of dealing with this problem.

17. The concept of loss is a central one in relation to the aetiology of many depressive illnesses. What are the significant losses commonly associated with growing old?

18. Mr John F., aged 67, has been depressed for six months. He has been admitted to your unit following an overdose of amitriptyline two days ago. He is now depressed, anxious and agitated with bizarre hypochondriacal ideas and ideas of unworthiness. Dietary intake is poor, insomnia is troublesome and the risk of suicide is considered high. Using the following evaluative list of this patient's needs, develop a nursing care programme.

PROBLEM	NURSING CARE
Protection from self-destructive impulses.	
Increasing self-esteem, confidence and optimism.	
Rest and relax.	
Reduce hypochondriacal thinking.	
Physical needs (diet, hygiene, sleep).	
Adjustment to developmental changes.	

19. Select a patient on your unit with puerperal depression, or use the following case-summary to complete the assigned work.

Janet D., aged 22, has been married four years and has recently given birth to her first child. Since being home from hospital Janet has felt increasingly tired, depressed and unable to cope. The baby is not feeding well and is fretful, keeping her awake most nights. Janet says she has never felt any real love for the child and this makes her feel guilty. To make matters worse her relationship with her husband has been under a strain due to Janet's disinclination to resume their sexual relationship. She wonders whether he really wanted the baby as they had become so accustomed to living a free and full life.

The crisis comes one night when the baby won't stop crying. Janet picks the baby up, shakes it violently and throws it into the cot. On admission Janet is depressed, anxious and tearful. She says she is not a real mother and would be better off dead.

i. Where such facilities exist mother and baby are often admitted together. What are the advantages and disadvantages of this arrangement?

ii. Develop a nursing care programme for Janet, indicating how you might help her achieve a satisfactory adjustment to her new role.

20. Mrs Dora C., aged 57, has been a patient on your ward for seven months. This is the longest spell she has had in hospital, but there is a history of admissions for bouts of depression, stretching back over 15 years. Dora does get quite depressed from time to time, but she is at best a rather helpless, dependent, self-absorbed lady, who has very little self-confidence. Her husband, who was quite supportive, died seven years ago, since when her admissions have increased in frequency. She has a small well-furnished house which she is reluctant to give up. As the community nurse assigned to care for this patient outline a programme of care to meet her needs.

MANIA

Mania (hypomania) is a term used to describe a pathological state of excitement characterised by elation and psychomotor overactivity. Although recurrent hypomania with no apparent depressive phases occurs, it is often encountered in manic-depressive psychosis, a condition in which the mood alternates between pathological depression and excitement.

The association between depression and mania is very close. Even during a manic phase, depressive symptoms may suddenly and fleetingly break through. Many authorities regard mania as a defensive reaction to the ego-threatening experience of guilt and self-deprecation common in depression. This would appear logical in the face of the egotistical ideas and unrealistic sense of well-being experienced by most manic patients.

21. John G., aged 28, and a clerical officer with the Inland Revenue, has been admitted to your ward in an acute hypomanic state. On admission he is very restless and appears quite unable to relax. He talks rapidly and disjointedly on a succession of topics and says he cannot stay long as he has important Government business in America to attend to. He laughs loudly at his own puns and appears very sensitive to the ward environment. When asked by the nurse to undress ready for a physical examination he suggests that she should also take off her clothes. John reacts very angrily when the doctor recommends that he should stay in hospital for a while. He says he has never felt fitter in his life and has far too many important things to attend to.

i. Make a list of the clinical features of hypomania highlighted in the above account
ii. Using the following problem-evaluation list, develop a nursing care plan for this patient.

PROBLEM	NURSING APPROACH
Needs to discharge energy and ideas.	
Reacts angrily to frustration.	
Lacks normal social restraint and inhibition and judgement.	
Delusional thought-content of a grandiose nature.	
Neglect of physical needs (diet, hygiene, rest).	
Over-responsive to environmental stimuli.	

Care of the patient with suicidal tendencies

Suicidal behaviour is considered here because of its relationship with depression. It is a term often used to embrace all acts of self-injury or poisoning, but it is important to realise that the motivation for such an act may be other than the wish to die. The intent, whether conscious or unconscious, may be to punish others; to draw attention to social difficulties and unhappiness or to provide temporary relief from emotional or physical pain. This does not mean that people who injure themselves for these motives are any less deserving of our concern and emotional support. We must try and appreciate the sense of isolation and desperation that so often precedes such acts, and although the manipulative 'appeal' effect of some such behaviour may be transparently clear to others it is not always so to the patient. A further point for consideration is that many acts with intentions other than self-destruction end tragically in suicidal accidents. The following is a useful classification of acts of self-injury.

A. *Fully intended acts*
   Suicide; Attempted suicide

B. *Acts with other intentions* (Parasuicide)
   Suicidal gesture; Suicidal accident.

The cause of suicidal behaviour is complex and many factors appear to contribute. We have already commented on the relationship between various psychiatric disorders and suicide, e.g. depression and alcoholism, in which aggressive, destructive feelings are turned inward towards self. You may find it helpful to refer again to the units dealing with these topics.

Although the suicide rate in the U.K. appears to be falling the number of parasuicides continues to rise. It is estimated that there are something like 60,000 suicidal gestures in the U.K. annually. A growing number of these are in the 15- to 20-year-old age group and a large proportion are young women. The most common injuries amongst this group are wrist lacerations or overdoses – usually of tranquillisers or analgesics. Often the act is carried out in the presence of others or where the individual is almost certain to be discovered.

The motivation for such acts is often to draw attention to the individual's frustration and unhappiness; to arouse concern and to change the behaviour of others. Often in the background there is a history of recent disagreements with parents, school difficulties, broken relationship with boy-friend, etc. Others are rather aimless, inadequate, 'impotent' people who learn to gain some relief by expressing their frustrations and tensions in this way.

You will find it helpful at this point to refer to the section on attention-seeking behaviour where the management of such patients is discussed.

22. Below is a list of other factors which appear to influence the individual's potential for suicide. Discuss each of these briefly:

Age	Social integration	Cultural background
Sex	Employment/financial status	Family history
Class	Religious affiliation	Seasonal variation

23. Durkheim, in his study 'Le Suicide', held the view that the source of suicidal behaviour lay in the coercive nature of social influences. He distinguished three types of suicide according to the type of disturbance in the relationship between society and the individual. Briefly discuss each of these categories and give an example of each.

i. Altruistic
ii. Egoistic
iii. Anomic

Many psychoanalysts, including Freud and Adler, have postulated an innate aggressive drive which becomes perverted during development and is expressed in self-destructive impulses. Karl Menninger, in his book *Man Against Himself*, interprets many forms of social deviance as being expressions of this self-destructive drive. Drug and alcohol-addiction, some automobile accidents, self-mutilation and asceticism are seen as examples of this. It is of interest that many who subscribe to this innate-drive theory stress lack of love in childhood as being a potent factor in its perversion.

24. Using your knowledge of the factors in causation write a descriptive profile of the type of person most likely to attempt suicide.

25. Following a suicide attempt there is often a significant and spontaneous improvement in mood and morale. What reasons can you give to explain this phenomenon?

26. The protection of patients with high risks rating from their self-destructive impulses is an important psychiatric nursing skill. Central to this skill is the ability to observe and recognise behavioural cues to suicidal acts. Warnings of suicidal intentions are usually given either in an overt or covert way, and if they can be recognised and appropriately responded to, fatal consequences could often be avoided.

List the features of a patient's speech/thought content and behaviour that would lead you to suspect him to be at risk.

Occasionally serious depressive illness may be masked by a superficial overlay of cheerfulness and purposefulness – the 'smiling depressive'. The nurse should not be misled by this superficial façade which is an attempt to cope with feelings of despair, guilt and self-reproach by keeping mentally and physically busy. However, during inactive, quieter moments these feelings may forcefully break through and a suicide attempt may be made.

27. It is important that the nurse should also be aware of signs of recovery. What factors indicated in the account below would suggest a suicide attempt is now unlikely?

June S. has been receiving in-patient treatment for a severe depressive illness. Coming on duty you find June in an angry mood. On regaining her composure she explains that she feels frustrated at having to remain in hospital for a further fortnight. She says she is anxious to return to work as this is a very busy time of the year at the store where she works and there is the possibility of promotion.

28. In addition to careful observation the management of at-risk patients should involve some degree of environmental control. This includes the removal of potentially dangerous articles (razor blades, manicure sets, dressing gown cords, matches, etc.), and restrictions of the patient's movement (confined to bed, to the day room, clothes removed, etc.) Many authorities believe it is unhelpful to apply these measures too strictly.

Discuss the possible reasons for this view.

A more positive approach in our view is for the nurse to engage in a therapeutic relationship with the patient, if necessary explaining that she is going to spend the next few hours with him because of the concern felt for his safety. This approach makes the need for strict environmental control unnecessary and makes close yet unobtrusive observation possible. Some patients are greatly reassured by this approach as they often feel confused and 'out of control'. Contact with the nurse also provides the opportunity for the release of tensions and for sharing underlying problems. Many patients feel a sense of remorse and guilt following a suicide attempt and acceptance of their behaviour and the genuine interest of the nurse can do much to dispense this feeling.

A few patients are so seriously disturbed that they repeatedly attempt to act upon their self-destructive urges. Such patients may be more safely nursed in seclusion and specialled by the nurse who should never in any circumstances leave the patient unsupervised.

29. Select a patient on your ward with suicidal tendencies. Describe how you have been able to use your relationship with this patient in a therapeutically helpful way.

30. It is unfortunate but true that suicidal gestures as a behavioural expression of unhappiness or frustration are learned by many susceptible individuals through the process of identification and reinforcement whilst in hospital. Explain the meaning of this statement and suggest ways in which it may be avoided.

31. Discuss the role of the following in the prevention of suicide:

i. Samaritans
ii. Crisis Intervention Service
iii. The community/neighbourhood
iv. Prescription, packaging and sale of drugs
v. Crisis Centres attached to Accident and Emergency departments.

NURSING THE DEPRESSED PATIENT
Self-Evaluation Test

1. Select from the list below *four* clinical features of depression:

a. amnesia;
b. poor concentration;
c. auditory hallucinations;
d. anorexia;
e. guilt feelings;
f. thought blocking;
g. insomnia;
h. disorientation.

2. Select from the list below *three* clinical features of hypomania:

a. Elation;
b. visual hallucinations;
c. confabulation;
d. restlessness;
e. grandiose ideas;
f. depersonalisation.

3. You are assigned to nurse a seriously depressed patient. In *Most* cases would you:

a. try and cheer her up by being bright and cheerful;
b. make her join in with others;
c. sit with her and try and be comforting and encouraging;
d. tell her she must try and snap out of it?

4. Which *three* of the following may be regarded as cues to suicidal behaviour:

a. morbid thought pattern;
b. overactivity;
c. retardation;
d. aggressiveness;
e. increasing social withdrawal;
f. concealing potentially dangerous items;
g. persecutory ideas?

5. The severely depressed patient is most likely to make a suicide attempt during the recovery phase. This is because:

a. the patient's hormone levels begin to increase;
b. the patient becomes frustrated by the restrictions of the hospital;
c. patients are unsupervised for longer periods at this time;
d. the patient's motivation and insight returns.

6. Select from the alternatives listed below the approach *most* helpful in the management of a hypomanic patient:

a. divert energy and attention to various low-key activities;
b. channel energy into organising social event for the unit;
c. seclude the patient until manic phase has subsided;
d. encourage vigorous physical exercise.

7. In most cases the reason why a manic patient does not take an adequate diet is . . . (Select the most appropriate response from the list below).

a. he believes food to be poisoned;
b. he believes he has some obstruction in his bowels;

c. he cannot sit still and concentrate long enough to eat;
d. his appetite is poor.

8. A depressed patient tells you that she is no good to anyone and deserves to be punished. Select the best reply from the list below:

a. it's silly to talk that way, you know it's not true;
b. you feel you are no good;
c. we have all done things we regretted later;
d. stop worrying about it and come and help me lay tables for tea.

Assertion and reason

Each of the questions in this section consists of an assertion followed by a reason. Assign to each question one of the five categories (a–e) given in the key below:

KEY

a. The assertion and reason are both true.
The reason is a correct explanation of the assertion.
b. The assertion and reason are both true.
The reason is *not* a correct explanation of the assertion.
c. The assertion is true but the reason is false.
d. The assertion is false but the reason is true.
e. The assertion and reason are both false.

ASSERTION

1. In cases of puerperal depression, bringing the baby into hospital with the mother is a helpful step.

REASON

Nursing staff can take over responsibility for the care of the baby throughout the mother's stay in hospital.

ASSERTION

2. The depressed patient who appears reasonably active, energetic and is able to smile is not seriously depressed.

REASON

Depressive feelings and thoughts may be temporarily suppressed by keeping physically and mentally active.

ASSERTION

3. Although at opposite poles of the mood spectrum, the association between mania and depression is very close.

REASON

Mania is an ego-defence reaction to depressive feelings and thoughts.

ASSERTION

4. There is often a rapid improvement in mood and optimism following an unsuccessful suicide.

REASON

Pent-up tensions are released and the support of relatives and friends rallied.

ASSERTION

5. In the care of depressed patients, occupational activities should not be demanding and should provide the patient with a sense of achievement.

REASON

Rest and relaxation are the most important facets of treatment.

ASSERTION

6. Maintaining strict observation and control in the care of suicidal patients is not always the most helpful approach.

REASON

A degree of privacy and freedom of movement should be respected as a basic human right.

ASSERTION

7. Depressive illness is quite common during the middle years of life.

REASON

The stress of modern life drains the emotional reserves of the individual.

ASSERTION

8. In the care of hypomanic patients a stimulating and social ward environment is most helpful.

REASON

Sensory receptiveness to the environment is blunted in hypomania.

True/False items

1. A depressed patient may refuse meals because he believes he cannot pay for them. (True; False)
2. In severe depression insomnia takes the form of difficulty in getting off to sleep. (True; False)
3. A person who says he is going to kill himself seldom does. (True; False)
4. Poor adjustment to a maternal role is an important causative factor in puerperal depression. (True; False)
5. Suicide is most common during the winter months. (True; False)
6. Suicidal gestures can often be learned from others as a means of gaining attention or relieving tension. (True; False)
7. Flight of ideas describes speech that moves rapidly and disjointedly from one topic to another. (True; False)
8. The egoistic suicide is suicide that occurs because the individual has tenuous links with society. (True; False)

REFERENCES AND FURTHER READING

Altschull, A. (1978), *Psychiatric Nursing*, Ballière Tindall.
Crowcroft, A. (1967), *The Psychotic*, Pelican.
Dalton, K. (1978), *Once a Month*, Fontana.
Durkheim, E. (1952), 'Le Suicide'.
Hilgard, R., Atkinson, R. C. and Atkinson, R. L. (1975), *Introduction to Psychology*, 6th edition, Harcourt Brace Jovanovich.
Menninger, K. (1938), *Man Against Himself*.
Mereness, D. (1978), *Essentials of Psychiatric Nursing*, Mosby.
Mitchell, A. (1975), *Depression*, Pelican.
Parker, G. (1978), *The Bonds of Depression*, Angus & Robertson.
Parkes, C. M. (1972), *Bereavement*, Pelican.
Rycroft, C. (1970), *Anxiety and Neurosis*, Pelican.
Sim, M. (1974), *Guide to Psychiatry*, Churchill Livingstone.
Stengal, I. (1973), *Suicide and Attempted Suicide*, Pelican.

Unit 4

Nursing the Anxious Patient

INTRODUCTION

Man is both blessed and cursed with a biological system that arouses and alerts him when his well-being is threatened. At a certain point this state of arousal is perceived as being unpleasant and is called anxiety. Such a system has served us well through our evolution, alerting us to danger and preparing us to take action against the hazards of our environment.

Today, however, man is faced with new hazards; new threats to his physical well-being, against many of which he finds it difficult to take immediate action. The afflictions of modern man, such as cancer and heart disease, the ever-present threat of nuclear war, growing urban street violence, noise, pollution; all represent stressful elements of modern life against which it is difficult to act. If threats to our physical well-being have changed, then certainly threats to our psychological well-being have increased and like many of the threats mentioned above they are often difficult to resolve. Loneliness, unhappy relationships, unemployment are examples of common stresses from which it is difficult to escape. It is often these chronic enduring stresses, as much as major stress events such as marital breakdown or bereavement, that undermine emotional reserves. Because of the stressful nature of modern society we should not be surprised that anxiety states are the most common of all mental health problems.

Anxiety should not, however, always be regarded as abnormal when it occurs; indeed as our opening statement suggests, anxiety is a useful and desirable human characteristic. Anxiety acts as a spur, prompting us to seek solutions to our difficulties; it 'keys us up' physically and mentally, enabling us to deal more effectively with day-to-day problems. People often work better under stress; but there are limits, and beyond a certain point anxiety begins to impair efficiency.

This unit aims to increase your understanding of the nature and causes of unhelpful, pathological anxiety and the effects it may have on the behaviour and general health of the individual. The unit also aims to develop your skills in caring for the anxious patient.

Much anxiety results from disharmony within our personal relationships and particularly from within the family; for it is through these close social bonds that we gain comfort and security and meet our sexual and emotional needs. The modern nuclear family is a very insular unit and frustrations and tensions which inevitably arise are often internalised and allowed to 'fester' and grow, further aggravating the situation and causing much unhappiness. It is possible that such tensions would once have been shared and resolved within the supporting context of an extended family network. Marital problems are occurring with increasing frequency. This is partly because people are marrying earlier and having their families earlier, often before they have the maturity to cope with these responsibilities; but also because the companionship element in the marital relationship has assumed more importance than ever before. People are not prepared to put up with defects in a relationship that has to span perhaps 50 years, and in an 'instant' age often expect 'instant' success and are less inclined to work towards building a successful and satisfying relationship. These factors, along with changing social and religious attitudes and the improved social and economic position of women, have made the stress of separation and divorce a common experience.

1. What are the problems most likely to be encountered during the first five years of marriage?

Sexual difficulties, despite our permissive and enlightened age, are still a common source of anxiety. Such problems often arise in early adolescence, in the early years of marriage and during middle age. Guilt feelings, fears about sexual adequacy or normality, frigidity and impotence can often underlie and be made worse by anxiety. (See Unit 10.)

Financial stresses also often contribute to anxiety, as people are seduced by modern selling techniques and the need to compete with each other for the material symbols of success, to over-stretch their incomes. Work stresses sometimes arise as the result of modern production processes which often create a monotonous and unfulfilling work situation. Others get caught up in a career structure that promotes them above their level of competence, exposing them to more responsibility than they are equipped to cope with. Many more women these days, because of personal or economic needs, attempt to hold down a full-time job and also run a home. This may work well in a situation where domestic responsibility is shared, but this is often not the case and coping with the demands of two often conflicting roles can undermine emotional reserves.

2. What aspects of your job make you feel most anxious?

This brief resumé of contemporary social stress points gives only part of the picture. While it is true that we all have our breaking point, some people are more emotionally resilient than others and are therefore less likely to become anxious in the face of such pressures.

Some people are inherently anxious, highly strung and sensitive, often reacting badly to the stresses of life. Others have a pervasive sense of personal inadequacy so that life to them in so many of its aspects is a trial. Others seem to lack the capacity to 'rise above' stress and seem easily overwhelmed by the frustrations and adversities of life, a difficulty exacerbated by our culture which discourages emotional expression, allowing anxieties to be bottled up rather than released and shared.

Some authorities regard such anxiety as resulting from childhood conflicts which have been repressed into the unconscious part of the mind. It is said these conflicts involve such things as aggressive, hostile feelings, felt by the child towards its parents. A conflict is thus set up in the child's mind; as they feel angry towards the person they depend on for their physical and emotional needs and can't risk losing. Such conflicts generate anxiety which is repressed but may later be reactivated by stresses, and as the repressive mechanism breaks down it gains conscious expression.

3. A warm, secure, loving relationship between a child and its parents in early life is the best insurance policy against anxiety there is.

Discuss this statement, indicating how difficulties the early mother–child relationship may arise and generate anxiety.

An alternative view of anxiety is that it arises as a learned response to specific situations in early life and then becomes generalised. For example a child may learn to feel afraid of his morose, austere father and that fear may become generalised to all authority figures, so that the individual is unreasonably apprehensive in his relationships with his teachers, senior colleagues, etc. A child frightened by a dog may as the result learn to be fearful not only of dogs but of all furry animals.

Whatever the origins of anxiety it is often most apparent at certain points during the developmental stages of life: adolescence, marriage, parenthood, middle age and old age. It is at these points in our lives that adjustments have to be made to our changing physical and psychological abilities and to new social circumstances. It is during these periods that many of the stresses we have been discussing tend to occur.

4. Describe the possible psychological and social difficulties with which the following individuals may be faced:
   i. A 23-year-old woman with an 18-month-old daughter who is separated from her husband
   ii. A 67-year-old widow whose husband died six months ago
   iii. A 48-year-old man with two teenage boys who is now unlikely to progress further in his career.

5. Try and recall a recent situation in which you felt anxious. Make a list of the physical sensations you experienced. What other reactions are known to occur?

   i. How are the physiological reactions associated with anxiety brought about and what functions do they serve?

An anxiety state is said to exist when anxiety becomes excessive and inappropriate, given the patient's circumstances. Individuals may experience fatigue and feel tense, irritable and on edge all the time. Their concentration is usually poor and their sleep may be restless, perhaps disturbed by unpleasant dreams. The anxious person is often troubled by various physical symptoms such as dyspepsia, diarrhoea, headaches and muscular aches and pains. He may also experience palpitations, sweating, tremors and dizzy spells. Anxiety impairs sexual performance and women may develop amenorrhoea. Sometimes the anxiety will become centred around one of these physical sensations and as a result the patient becomes morbidly hypochondriacal, thinking he has heart disease or cancer of the stomach. Very often the person has no clear idea of why he is anxious and is unaware of the relationship between his emotional discomfort and physical state. Once physical pathology has been ruled out a simple explanation of this relationship (by the doctor or the nurse) can be greatly reassuring. Occasionally acute panic attacks occur, during which the patient's heart races, he hyperventilates, shakes and sweats profusely. Often the experience is so profound that the person thinks he is going to die.

Sometimes anxiety takes a more specific form and is associated with certain situations or objects, so that the person seeks to avoid these whenever possible. This is called phobic anxiety and is very common in the general population. Many people have unreasonable fears of moths, blood, crowds, etc., but are able to keep their anxiety under control. This is not always the case, however, and some people suffer excessive anxiety in certain situations and become socially disabled as the result. Agoraphobia is a common phobia in which people feel overwhelmed by anxiety when they attempt to leave their homes. Social phobia occurs frequently, in which people are acutely anxious in the presence of others, particularly strangers, and gradually become more and more reclusive. School phobia is again quite common and generally arises in children who feel unsure in their relationship with mother and feel if they are not with her all the time they may lose her.

Patients suffering from anxiety states seldom require admission to hospital and can usually be treated in the community setting. However, anxiety is a common and normal reaction to hospitalisation and the stress of illness, whether of a psychiatric or medical nature. Nurses need therefore to be aware of patients' anxiety and take steps to reduce stress as much as possible.

6. With reference both to your own experience of being a patient in hospital and your observations of patients' reactions, complete the following rating scale. Compare and discuss your results with your set.

Which of the following are generally found most distressing by patients in hospital:

	Neutral	Very distressing
Admission to hospital		
Having an injection		
Night-time in hospital		
Having a bath with the nurse helping		
Talking to the consultant		
Having to talk about your illness		
Sister's day off		
Boredom		
Being away from the family		
Noise		
Being away from your job		
Seeing other patients who are very ill		

	Neutral	Very distressing
The ward routine		
Your illness		
Anticipating a treatment or procedure		
Visiting time		
Using the commode		
Using the bed pan		
The nurse's report		
Being discharged		
Talking to the nurses		
Being a 'patient'		
Knowing your relatives are talking to the nursing staff.		

7. Discuss the ways in which the patient's experience of those items which have a high stress rating can be improved.

8. You have been assigned to supervise Mr John C., aged 28, who is due to have the first treatment of a course of ECT later that morning. John appears very tense, anxious and preoccupied.
   Outline your approach to the care of this patient.

It should be remembered that people in hospital do not always express their anxiety in overt ways we have described. Some may appear withdrawn and distracted, preoccupied with private fantasies; for in this way many people are able to cope with distressing circumstances. Sometimes anxious patients may become unusually aggressive or easily irritated while others seem 'buoyantly confident' and cheerful, a reaction which appears out of place in their current circumstances. Other patients may behave in regressive and dependent ways, seeking to gain security by adopting child-like behaviour.

It is important that nurses are prepared to take time talking and listening to their patients. They should appear available and approachable and should try, in their contacts with patients, to foster a sense of confidence and security. It is greatly reassuring to be able to share your worries with someone who understands and is concerned. Simply talking-out your problems can help relieve tensions and also helps people to see their difficulties in a clearer and more realistic way. Often it is appropriate for the nurse to give information and advice, or for social workers to intervene in a practical way; but in many cases the patient should be given the encouragement and support to seek their own solutions to their difficulties. You may find it helpful at this point to refer to Unit 2, where the nature of reassurance is discussed.

Activities of a recreational or occupational nature are useful as they may help ease away tensions, displace anxiety and prevent the patient becoming morbidly preoccupied with his problems. Vigorous activities such as badminton and dancing, or quieter activities conducted in a social atmosphere, such as painting, craft-work, or nature rambles may be helpful. Board games, listening to music, and reading are all useful unwinders.

9. Make a list of the ways in which you are able to unwind and displace your frustrations and anxieties.

In addition to supportive counselling many patients may benefit from participation in specific forms of therapeutic activity. Relaxation techniques can be taught which, when some degree of proficiency has been achieved, can be applied to everyday situations so that a more relaxed approach to life is encouraged. Progressive relaxation of muscles is learned first of all, followed by controlled breathing techniques and finally mental exercises, all of which combine to produce a state of real relaxation.

Group therapy provides the opportunity for patients to share and explore their problems with others who may have similar difficulties in a supporting and accepting atmosphere. Group discussion may be combined with psycho-drama exercises, perhaps simulating family situations which are a significant part of a patient's problem. Social-skills training may be a valuable group activity to build up assertiveness and social confidence, and Gestalt exercises may be usefully employed with patients whose primary problem is anxiety. Some patients with anxiety states may have specific underlying marital or sexual problems and would benefit from conjoint therapy or sex therapy.

10. Write outline notes on any of the forms of treatment mentioned above.

Behaviour therapy techniques have recently proved very helpful in the treatment of phobic anxiety, and nurses are increasingly playing an active part in such treatment. The most useful techniques currently being employed are systematic desensitisation and modelling.

Systematic desensitisation is a form of counter-conditioning in which the relaxation response is encouraged in situations which formerly evoked acute anxiety. In this way maladaptive behaviour (anxiety and avoidance) when confronted, say by a cat, can be weakened and extinguished by strengthening an antagonistic response (relaxation). Patients are first of all taught relaxation techniques and then exposed to situations which they find stressful and have previously avoided. Usually the sessions start with the situations the patient finds least difficult, and as they begin to feel confident and relaxed the next most difficult is tried until the final target has been reached. During therapy sessions the phobic situations encountered may be visually imagined or real – the therapist encouraging the patient to relax, using the techniques taught, throughout the exposure.

This can be combined with modelling which makes use of the process of identification. Here the therapist carries out some action that the patient finds difficult, for example cuddling a cat, and encourages the patient to join her. The therapist appears confident and relaxed in the situation and this confidence is transferred to the patient. The patient is given support and encouragement to carry out the feared activity along with the therapist and given praise and approval for successes.

11. Mrs Penny W., aged 40, has been admitted to your unit for treatment of her phobic anxiety. Penny has been virtually housebound for the past two years. She has always felt a certain amount of tension and apprehension when travelling any distance from her home, but recently even going to the corner shop made her feel very anxious. Penny would like to be able to walk in her local park like she used to; travel into town for shopping and entertainment and travel the eight miles by bus to a nearby village to visit her daughter. It has been agreed that these should be the targets of her treatment while in hospital.

Describe how systematic desensitisation and modelling might be employed in the treatment of this patient.

12. Philip Y., aged 17, has been admitted to your unit with a history of hypochondriacal anxiety and panic attacks. Philip has always been rather shy and reserved and known as a 'worrier'. Philip recently started work and was ridiculed by his work mates for having a small penis. This aggravated feelings he already had about whether he was normal as he masturbated quite a lot and worried that all his workmates seemed to have had sexual experience and he hadn't. His recent attempts at 'seduction' had met with a rejection and Philip has become convinced he is abnormal and that girls find him unattractive.

Mrs Teresa A., aged 70, is an intelligent, active lady with a pleasant though rather reserved and sensitive disposition. Mrs A.'s husband died five months ago and since then she has lived alone. She has two married daughters who live locally and call in on their mother frequently. Recently Mrs A. has become rather morbidly preoccupied with illness. She complains of dyspepsia, nausea and diarrhoea and despite her GP's assurance to the contrary she believes she has cancer. She is now sleeping badly and is afraid of being on her own. On occasions she has had acute episodes of anxiety when she shakes, sweats profusely, hyperventilates, and on one such occasion fainted. Although Mrs A. coped well with the initial stress of losing her husband she has since found it difficult to set her life in motion again. Most of her interests and friends were shared with her husband and she says she feels conscious of everything being an 'anniversary': 'I'm constantly aware that the last time I did this or went there he was with me'. This has made Mrs A. feel increasingly lonely and insecure.

As the nurse assigned to care for Philip Y. and Teresa A. outline your approach, indicating how you would reduce general anxiety and help facilitate a better adjustment.

NURSING THE OBSESSIONAL PATIENT

Obsessional behaviour may be seen as a form of protection against anxiety. In its extreme form it presents either as elaborate compulsive rituals or as alien thoughts of a persistent and intrusive nature. Such behaviour can be extremely disabling and distressing both for the sufferer and his family. Most of us behave in mildly obsessional ways from time to time. We check and re-check to make sure we have locked the door securely, or switched the lights or the cooker off; we are aware that our behaviour is excessive but we cannot feel at ease until we have carried it out. Many of us feel uneasy if our routine is upset or our homes untidy. In some people such characteristics are the central and dominating features of their personalities. They are described as having an obsessional personality.

13. Write a descriptive profile of an imaginary person with an obsessional personality, indicating what her/his domestic and occupational life might be like.

The origins of such behaviour are obscure but are said to lie in early development. Many experts see obsessional behaviour as resulting from excessively strict parental attitudes towards socialisation and sexuality. For example, the mother over-anxious to toilet train her child may consistently scold and punish him for soiling himself. Children exposed to such attitudes may grow up with the notion that making a mess is dirty and bad and that controlling themselves, being clean and tidy, brings approval. Such ideas can become associated with emotional and sexual development. It can be seen how the morally strict, emotionally controlled, highly organised and orderly person emerges out of this.

Clearly having such a personality can have advantages, particularly in certain occupations such as banking; but when these traits are excessive they may become restrictive, preventing the individual living easily and happily with others and from enjoying his life to the full. Obsessional personality traits enable the individual to exercise maximum control over his life. It reduces the element of chance – the likelihood of the unexpected or spontaneous occurring. By controlling the events of his day-to-day life so rigidly and by repressing his feelings he is able to keep anxiety at bay.

Obsessional disorders occur when this control begins to break down. Events may occur which disorganise his life; for example redundancy, illness, marital difficulties; or his ability to repress unconscious feelings and drives may begin to fail. The individual attempts to deal with the mounting anxiety and guilt by increasing the strictness and thoroughness of his routine. Gradually compelling and disruptive rituals begin to emerge which commonly take the form of checking or washing rituals. He may spend hours in the bathroom attending to his dress and hygiene, or perhaps feel the need to get up several times in the night to check the window catches or light switches and plug sockets. He realises his behaviour is irrational but feels compelled by mounting tensions and the notion that if the ritual is not carried out some mishap will befall him or his family. Rituals tend to be self-reinforcing as the person is rewarded for performing the ritual by a fall in anxiety and tension. A vicious circle is often created in that ritualising generates its own anxiety which increases the need to ritualise. Some authorities see the patients' rituals as a form of atonement for feelings of guilt.

Obsessional thoughts are characterised by their intrusive and persistent nature. People may have recurring thoughts about stabbing their partner or children, or be troubled by blasphemous or obscene thoughts totally foreign to their nature. Such ideas do not represent true intent, but are symbolic of over-repressed feelings and drives perhaps of a sexual or aggressive nature. They may be extremely distressing to, and so dominate, the individual's consciousness that concentration and efficiency are impaired.

Obsessional behaviour is often such an ingrained feature of a person's personality and way of life that to expect radical change in response to therapy is unrealistic. The severity of their behaviour does fluctuate with their life's circumstances and much can be done to help them through difficult periods and to modify their personalities so that excessive ritualising is less likely in the future.

Patients are often reluctant to come into hospital because they are afraid they will be prevented from following their rituals through or that they will be regarded with derision. Their rituals are often elaborate and time-consuming, disrupting the fabric of their day so that meals are missed, work is difficult, sleep is lost and the routine of others is interfered with. Their behaviour may be seen as absurd and unnecessary and the nurse may be tempted to hurry the patient along, to be disapproving or to prevent rituals being carried out. Such an approach will only serve to increase the patient's anxiety and tensions; resulting in increase in the patient rituals or provoking an acute panic attack. In the relatively calm and orderly atmosphere of the hospital ward and away from demands of his normal day-to-day life the patient's obsessional symptoms may begin to subside and become less disabling and disruptive. The nurse should do all she can to make the person feel accepted, secure and relaxed. Diversional and displacement activities of an occupational and recreational nature are useful. It may be helpful to review any underlying problems with the patient, although it should be kept in mind that exposing such difficulties may have the effect of increasing anxiety and ritualistic behaviour. Counselling of this nature should only be carried out under the direction of the psychiatrist. Care should be taken to ensure the patient's general health does not suffer.

The treatment team must decide on the best approach to the patient's obsessional behaviour. In some cases time limits on rituals may be set to make the patient's routine more controlled and acceptable. This is done gradually and fully discussed with the patient and his co-operation gained. Anxiety is reduced in other ways – drugs such as chlordiazepoxide (Librium) or chlormipramine (Anafranil) have proved useful. The latter drug has been found particularly helpful as depressive symptoms are not uncommon in obsessional states.

The nurse should be supportive and encouraging, helping the patient achieve a more acceptable schedule.

Recently behavioural techniques have proved valuable in the treatment of obsessional disorders, and nurses are increasingly playing a central role in such treatment under the guidance of the psychiatrist. The techniques most commonly employed are response prevention and modelling.

14. Mr John B., aged 36, is a patient on your unit suffering from an obsessional disorder. Going to bed has become a nightmare for John. It has frequently been 2 a.m. before he has been able to retire, by then exhausted, to bed. He has developed an elaborate checking ritual which involves checking all the window catches, door locks, plug sockets, light switches and taps a set number of times and in a given order. If his system gets out of sequence John feels compelled to start all over again. He becomes very agitated and tense and only begins to relax when he has completed his ritual.

Describe how response prevention and modelling might be employed in the treatment of this patient.

Patients who have obsessional ideas can be helped by the use of thought stopping techniques. Patients are taught relaxation and given an alternative idea to focus on when the obsession is particularly troublesome. Treatment, whether of a conventional or behavioural nature, may be carried out partly or wholly in the patient's home. As we have indicated it may be possible for the patient to reduce his rituals while in the orderly, supportive atmosphere of the hospital; but clearly patients need to gain some control over their obsessions in their own domestic environment. Elaborate obsessional behaviour often puts the family under considerable strain and they may need practical advice and assistance in developing helpful, supportive attitudes.

15. Cathy B., aged 30, has been admitted to your ward in a depressed and agitated state with a history of severe obsessional behaviour. Her rituals centre around her personal hygiene and have built up over the last two years and have now become quite disabling. Cathy has a dread that she will become contaminated with germs and will infect others. She showers and puts on a complete set of clean clothes every morning and during the course of the day may shower herself and change all her clothes again five or six times. Her discarded clothes have to be thoroughly washed often several times before she can wear them again. Cleaning the house, going to the toilet, going shopping are now very difficult as tension builds up and she feels compelled to carry out her ritual. She avoids as many people as she can and has recently not been able to touch or kiss her husband and children for fear of contaminating them.

Cathy has always been a strikingly neat and tidy person. She is methodical, likes everything in its place and even her relationships have a formal, regularised quality. Her rituals seem to date from the birth of her second baby, $2\frac{1}{2}$ years ago. Cathy admits she did not want the child.

Discuss the ways in which this patient might be helped by the community team emphasising the nursing involvement.

THE MANAGEMENT OF ATTENTION-SEEKING BEHAVIOUR

A great deal of disturbed and disturbing behaviour that the nurse meets with in her day-to-day work may be designed to arouse the concern and attention of others. It may take the form of excessive complaints or demands, bogus symptoms, negativism, helplessness, temper tantrums, food refusal, absconding, wrist-cutting, overdosing or window-smashing etc.

Attention-seeking behaviour such as this may essentially be a reflection of the patient's concern about his immediate circumstances. Most of us from time to time – when faced with personal difficulties, frustrations or illness – have behaved in regressive ways, seeking, although not being fully aware of our intentions, to gain the comfort and support of others. People in hospital, faced with the anxieties about their illness and treatment, separated from familiar sources of comfort and security, commonly behave in such ways. It should be remembered also that patients do not leave behind personal and social difficulties when they come into hospital. In fact such difficulties may be made considerably worse by hospitalisation. Marital tensions, worries about the children, financial difficulties and occupational problems may continue to preoccupy the patient and precipitate attention-seeking episodes.

16. Comment on any attention-seeking episodes you have encountered during recent clinical placements, indicating what the precipitating factors were and how the episodes were managed by the nursing team.

Attention-seeking, however, may sometimes be more pervasive than this and so colour the persons' behaviour that they are unable to achieve any real stability or satisfaction in their lives and relationships. People who behave in this way sometimes have a characteristic personality structure – the so-called hysterical personality. They are generally immature, egocentric, theatrical people whose demonstrative feelings lack depth and sincerity. Such people find it difficult to tolerate the frustrations and disappointments of everyday life and often over-react in the way we have described. They are suggestible people who are easily influenced by the behaviour and ideas of others. Some may be very demanding and manipulative in their relationships often taking a perverse delight in the distress and annoyance they cause, while others are quite ineffectual in their dealings with people and their relationships seldom amount to anything. Such people are clearly going to run into social difficulties and marital and sexual problems; drug and alcohol abuse and minor offences such as shoplifting are common amongst this group.

17. What do you consider the attributes of adult maturity?
In general terms what factors do you think have a key influence on the development of such attributes?

Closely allied to attention-seeking behaviour is the conversion reaction. Here the patient unconsciously adopts any one of an array of physical and mental symptoms. Conversion reactions commonly take the form of fits, amnesia, vomiting, paralysis, aphonia, etc. Such disabilities serve as a solution to some current personal crisis and have the added advantage of arousing the concern and attention of others. Careful investigation must be carried out to exclude physical pathology. Often the symptoms present as approximations of the illness and do not conform to the true medical presentation. Sometimes they have been suggested by illnesses the patient has recently read about or has seen in others. Some authorities suggest that in some cases the 'hysterical' presentation masks sub-clinical pathology and the illness later emerges. Another common feature is the lack of concern shown by many patients often in the face of serious disability. To the patient the symptoms are genuine and there is considerable resistance to any suggestion that the disorder is 'in the mind'. It should be remembered that the genesis of these disorders takes place below the level of conscious awareness and that the symptoms have a protective function. Giving up their symptoms would mean again being confronted with their difficulties and anxieties. Occasionally such people become so dependent on their symptoms that they become chronic invalids.

18. Briefly distinguish between conversion reactions, malingering, hypochondriasis and Munchausen's syndrome.

It has been suggested that people who regularly make use of attention-seeking behaviour to cope with stressful circumstances are people that have never felt valued, loved and lovable for themselves. In early life they never felt able legitimately to claim the attention of their parents. Gradually such individuals learn that by putting on an act, playing up, or by becoming 'sick' they are able to achieve some attention and recognition even if that attention takes the form of disapproval. Any attention is better than none at all. If such behaviour is reinforced by repeated experience it is likely to become a durable feature of the individual's personality. As he goes through life he may frequently retreat into the sick role or 'play up' whenever life becomes difficult or his relationships threatened. It will be clear that some forms of attention-seeking contain aggressive elements. This is said to represent traces of the unacceptable and therefore repressed hostility felt by the individual as a child towards its parents.

Whatever the origins of attention-seeking it is clear that the immediate circumstances of the patient can provoke and prolong such behaviour. An important factor here is the attitudes of the nursing staff which often become unsympathetic towards such patients. Nurses come to see such behaviour as being calculated and false and become increasingly irritated and annoyed by the patient, resulting in avoidance and unsatisfactory care. A relationships gap can easily open up between staff and the patient, creating further anxiety and insecurity and resulting in an increase in attention seeking.

19. Mrs Joyce D., aged 58, a widow, has been in hospital for four months with depression. Her prevailing attitude is one of hopelessness, helplessness and passivity. She requires a great deal of prompting, encouragement and support to manage even quite simple day-to-day tasks. Recently she has begun to behave 'hysterically', falling about, refusing meals, and displaying 'crazy' behaviour. The staff have become exasperated by what they see as her lack of effort to get well and her over-dependent attitudes.

At a staff meeting Nurse Steve M. puts forward the view that Joyce is swinging the lead and should be discharged. He feels that if she had to cope she would. Some of the staff agree with Steve; others take a different view of the situation.

Imagine you are a member of the ward team. What would your attitude towards this patient be and why?

Open discussion amongst staff about their feelings towards such patients is vital to ensure that their attitudes remain objective and the care they provide helpful. Staff should be prepared to support each other as such patients can be very trying and provocative to nurse. The approach to care must be fully understood by all members of the nursing team to ensure the care given is consistent.

The social atmosphere of the ward can do much to reduce attention seeking behaviour. It should be bright and clean and well organised; nurses should be seen as being accessible, approachable and efficient. It is important that the nurses have an awareness of the emotional discomfort of patients and are prepared to spend time listening, providing support and giving advice, or information where appropriate. Nurses should remember that many patients who are worried and distressed disguise their feelings and only express them in oblique ways such as by complaining excessively and unreasonably. It is also important that nurses do not over-react to demands, threats or emotional displays. Consistent, regular attention should be given, the nurse using her contact with the patient, both to be supportive and to firmly encourage mature responsible behaviour. Patients with conversion symptoms may become quite depressed and anxious as their symptoms subside, and require considerable reassurance and encouragement. The patient's day should be sensibly structured to include tasks and activities that encourage self-help and responsibility, prevent morbid self-absorption, help displace aggressive and anxious feelings and promote relaxation.

In the case of patients whose symptoms are more persistent and disruptive a therapeutic milieu that encourages personal growth and learning is essential. Participation in group therapy may give increasing awareness and understanding of their behaviour and its effect on others. They may find within the group an acceptance, recognition and support which may help them gradually to abandon their attention-seeking behaviour and conversion symptoms. Group pressure to conform to more acceptable and mature ways of behaving may also help modify behaviour. Within the group context they may learn to deal more effectively with people and cope with stress in less disruptive ways. Group therapy in which self-revelation, feedback and discussion are the principal activities may be supplemented by role-play exercises, projective art sessions, social-skills training and relaxation therapy.

As we have suggested it is clearly important that nurses do not reinforce regressive behaviour by over-reacting to attention-seeking episodes, and that mature and responsible behaviour should be encouraged and rewarded using positive reinforcers, such approval and privileges. Certain behaviour such as wrist-cutting or window-smashing cannot be ignored, but the nurse should try not to make an undue fuss of the patient or resort to punitive measures and should simply take whatever action is necessary to bring the situation under control in a quiet and efficient manner. This behavioural approach to general care should be applied as systematically and consistently as possible and ideally other patients in the unit should be aware of the need not to encourage deviant behaviour. Staff must define as clearly as possible what behaviour they will reward, for example being helpful and considerate to others, using time constructively, being open and honest in their conversation with others, being reliable, etc.

20. Using negative reinforcement in response to attention-seeking episodes, for example applying restrictions, withdrawal of privileges, isolating the patient, etc., seldom results in any significant improvement in behaviour and may have the opposite effect.

Discuss the reasons for this statement.

21. Patrick S., aged 26, has been referred to your unit for treatment as a condition of his probation. Patrick has a long history of overdosing, shop-lifting and vandalism. He is a single man of average intelligence and currently unemployed. Patrick is a very isolated young man who has great difficulty in sustaining relationships. He tends to be diffident and demanding and is given to bouts of melancholic self-pity. He cannot cope with frustrations, and attention-seeking episodes usually follow some upset with his mother or mounting frustration at his lack of adequacy with girls. He is very suggestible and has recently struck up an association with a group of drug-users; he has been experimenting with amphetamines and barbituarates. Patrick's widowed mother presents as a long-suffering martyr. She has tended to cling to and manipulate her two children over the years to meet her own emotional needs, and has never been able to give Patrick the confidence, security and self-regard he needs to assert his independence and deal effectively with others.

Identify the problems of the above patient and work out a programme of care you feel might help resolve his difficulties.

22. Alison H., aged 17, has been admitted to your ward following an overdose of paracetamol. This is the third time in the last six months that Alison has required admission for this reason. These episodes seem to follow some disagreement with 'Mum' or on this occasion being turned down for a job. The problem seems to be that Alison has never felt close to her mother. She feels she has always had to compete for her mother's attention with her younger sister and has always had to 'make' her mother take an interest. Alison's father died two years ago and recently Mrs H. has formed a close relationship with another man.

Alison does not seem to have a very 'generous' view of herself. She does not regard herself as a very capable, likeable or attractive person. She has 'terrific moods' which seem to be triggered off by any real or imagined rejection or failure in her life or by her own disparaging thoughts. She cannot understand how her mother could carry on with someone else so soon after her father's death.

Mrs H. says Alison has always been a difficult child. She had a difficult pregnancy and found the first few years of bringing Alison up to be a trial. Her husband wasn't very helpful or supportive and she suspected him of being unfaithful to her at this time. Mrs H. and Alison don't communicate a great deal and when they do it is often to row about clothes/make-up, stopping out and boy-friends. She feels Alison behaves in antagonistic and defiant ways just to upset her. She feels Alison is selfish and ungrateful. Mrs H. had a rather restricted youth and at a time when she feels the need to be seen as attractive and desirable, resents and feels threatened by youthful attractiveness, vitality and opportunity. She regards Alison's overdosing as 'silly and hysterical'.

i. Discuss your feelings towards patients like Alison who persistently overdose.

ii. Outline your approach to the psychological care of this patient during the admission period.

iii. How could this patient benefit from family therapy. Explore further the feelings and attitudes that could emerge in such sessions that might have contributed to Alison's behaviour

THE PSYCHOSOMATIC APPROACH TO PATIENT CARE

The term psychosomatic (mind–body) is used in two ways in medicine. First it is used in a general way to emphasise the close relationships between mind and body that exist both in health and disease. Secondly the term is used in a rather more narrow sense to describe a small group of illnesses, for example peptic ulcer, in which emotion is said to play a central part in either causing or exacerbating the illness.

We have described the mind-body relationships at work in several units of this book – the effect of depression on digestion, the role of anxiety in producing muscular pain and the confused behaviour that follows degenerative changes in the brain. This close relationship is again clearly evident in many medical disorders which are not in themselves of emotional origin. Cushing's disease, for example, is often accompanied by euphoric excitable behaviour, while thyrotoxicosis may result in behaviour that closely resembles acute anxiety. It is widely recognised that reactions to illness, response to treatment and recovery rates are closely related to the patient's emotional state and attitude; clearly a psychosomatic approach to the management of patients can have considerable benefit.

23. Tolerance of pain can be seen to vary considerably from one person to another. Consider how psychological and cultural factors may influence the level of tolerance.

What are the implications of your comments for the care of patients in pain?

24. Mrs Sally P. complains to her doctor that she has been feeling most unwell just lately and sometimes thinks she is 'losing her mind'. Sally says she feels tired, irritable and on edge all the time and that she keeps forgetting things. She also complains that she has been having a lot of headaches just recently and that her vagina has been very sore, preventing her carrying on her sex life. Since her periods stopped she has been having 'flushes' which she finds very embarrassing and is reluctant to go out socially because of them.

i. What practical advice and help can be given to women experiencing unpleasant menopausal symptoms?

ii. Comment on the usefulness of an out-patient 'menopausal group'.

25. A patient you are visiting in the community complains that she is having great difficulty in getting off to sleep at night. What could be the reason for this? What practical suggestions might you make to help solve this problem?

26. Consider the reasons why chemically non-active substances will sometimes have the same effect on symptoms as chemically active drugs (the placebo effect).

27. As life has become more and more sedentary, obesity has become a more common problem predisposing people to cardiovascular disease and diabetes. The fundamental cause of obesity is a continued excess of calorie intake over output. Psychological factors are also clearly important in the cause and management of obesity where overeating has provided some relief from feelings of frustration, insecurity, anxiety or boredom.
Outline a weight-reduction programme for an obese patient indicating how a psychological approach might help.

Earlier in the unit we noted the effects of emotional arousal on the body. It was seen that anxiety can have a considerable effect on heart rate, blood pressure, respiration etc., as well as producing more subtle changes in the blood chemistry through the action of adrenaline and cortisol. It should not surprise us therefore, that if states of emotional arousal are not relieved by action or expression and persist, that in time structural changes may occur in the organs and tissues of vulnerable individuals.

28. A widely accepted theory of how stress diseases arise is the 'stress adaptation syndrome' proposed by Hans Seyle. Briefly outline this theory.

The well-documented studies of Wolf and Wolf on their subject Tom illustrates well the impact of emotion on the organs and tissues of the body. Observation of Tom's stomach through a gastric fistula showed how anxiety, anger and resentment increased the motility, acid secretion and blood flow of the stomach. Patients with duodenal ulcers are often worrying, conscientious, frustrated people who have an overactive nerve supply to their stomachs. In such individuals the stomach empties rapidly, exposing the first part of the duodenum to imperfectly neutralised gastric juice. Ulcers commonly form on the mucosa of the first part of the duodenum. In gastric ulcers the process is rather different and excess amounts of hydrocholoric acid are not normally found. However, as studies like those on Tom have shown, the increased vascularity in emotional arousal may produce minor haemorrhages in the mucosa which form tiny ulcers that are exacerbated by the action of pepsin and hydrochloric acid.

Why specific parts of the body are vulnerable and others not remains unknown. It seems likely that some constitutional defect, either in the organ itself or in the nerve supply, is responsible.

29. Select a patient on your ward that you have nursed suffering from bronchial asthma. Write a brief clinical profile indicating how psychological factors are implicated.

Describe the nursing management of this patient, emphasising the psychological aspects of care.

Ulcerative colitis is another illness that has long been regarded as having an important emotional element. It is a recurring disorder characterised by severe diarrhoea, the stools frequently containing blood and mucus. Abdominal pain is often severe and the patient becomes weak, anaemic and emaciated. Like many psychosomatic disorders the illness is said to be associated with a particular personality type. Patients are often fussy, orderly, meticulous and rigid people. Certainly acute episodes of the illness commonly follow some stress experience such as leaving home or starting a new job. It is worth noting that the stress need not necessarily have unpleasant overtones – passing an examination or going on holiday may precipitate attacks.

Myocardial infarction has also often been associated with stress. Current ideas on causation do not support this view but nevertheless psychological factors are clearly important in the management of such patients. 'Coronary' patients often become depressed, anxious, dependent and inert following their illness and require much advice and support to encourage a more confident and active approach to life. Similarly stress has been implicated in the development of essential hypertension. Many hypertensive patients appear emotionally restrained people who have difficulty in expressing and discharging their frustrations and feelings. Chronic stress may be partly responsible for the thickening and narrowing of the arterial walls which is responsible for the persistent high blood pressure. Supportive counselling and advice to reduce the stress levels in their life, plus help to achieve a more relaxed approach to life through relaxation and biofeedback techniques, can prove a useful supplement to drug treatment for hypertension.

30. One of the most common disorders amongst the general population is headaches. Almost everyone suffers from one from time to time, and millions of pounds worth of analgesics are consumed in the UK every year for the relief of headache. Some people suffer chronic headaches, a small proportion of these people have some associated disorder such as hypertension which is responsible; the majority however have either vascular headaches of the migraine type or tension headaches, or a combination of the two.

i. Compare the symptoms of tension headache with those of migraine.
ii. How is stress and personality implicated in migraine?
iii. Discuss the treatment of migraine, indicating how behavioural therapy, biofeedback and relaxation techniques may help.

In our introduction to the unit on attention-seeking behaviour we mentioned food-refusal as a common attention-seeking ploy. Sometimes food-refusal may be prolonged and lead to extreme weight loss. When this occurs in the absence of physical pathology, particularly in adolescent girls, it is likely to be associated with a disorder called anorexia nervosa.

The characteristics of this disorder are a refusal and repugnance of food, extreme thinness, amenorrhoea and a distorted perception of body image. Anorexic patients see themselves as being much fatter than they in fact are. Patients with this disorder become preoccupied with their weight and worry incessantly about calories and how to avoid meals. Some may take regular laxatives; others go on food 'binges', eating until they vomit. In this way they achieve a sense of emptiness which gives them, for a time, peace of mind. Anorexic patients commonly employ 'decoy' behaviour to distract the attention and concern of others away from their weight loss. They may show a great interest in preparing and cooking food, reading cookery books or shopping for food. They may appear energetic and pad themselves out with layers of clothing to appear bigger than they really are. As the illness progresses it places many restrictions on their life, they may stop going out, having boy-friends, or pursuing their careers and studies.

The cause of anorexia remains uncertain. Some authorities see the disorder as an attempt to postpone or avoid the problems of coming to terms with a more adult social and sexual role. It seems that by postponing physical maturation the patient is able to retreat back into childhood dependency and regain the comfort and protection of parental care. Often the mothers of such patients have not proved to be very good role models, presenting sex as an unpleasant experience to be endured and their responsibilities as wife and mother as something of a trial. Other experts have emphasised such factors as marital tensions in the home, fashion, depression, examination pressures, teasing by family or friends about post-pubertal plumpness, as being important in the development of this disorder.

31. Discuss the adjustment difficulties and social pressures that might face a 15-year-old girl.

The treatment for anorexic patients usually involves strict nursing supervision, a behavioural element and counselling. The patient is nursed in bed, preferably in a single room, and is initially allowed up only to use the commode. In the early stages of treatment privileges such as visiting, radio, TV, favourite magazines, etc., are restricted. As target points on the weight progress chart are achieved the patient is allowed to spend more time up and allowed more visits, etc.

Meals must be supervised to prevent the patients hiding food or making themselves vomit. Nurses should not be taken in by complaints of headaches, stomach aches, or assurances that they will eat 'in a little while'. Small meals supplemented by calorific drinks are more acceptable to the patient in the early stages and as treatment progresses normal size meals of 3000 calories a day can be introduced. The nurse needs to be firm but also supportive, keeping in mind the patient's very real fear of putting on weight.

Patients need much encouragement and help to adopt a more accepting attitude towards their weight gain and body image. A weekly check should be carried out and a gain of about 3 lb is considered acceptable. Help should be given with any underlying emotional or personal problem, and family counselling can be helpful in cases where the emotional undercurrents at home and the parental relationship appear to be a significant factor in the illness. Relapses are not uncommon when the patient leaves hospital and is faced with living a more normal life style than the one they were accustomed to during their illness. Continued support by the community team may be useful.

32. Select a patient you have nursed suffering from anorexia nervosa.

i. Write a pro-clinical profile of this patient, highlighting the clinical features and general dieting behaviour of the patient.

ii. What factors do you feel have contributed to the development of the illness in your patient?

iii. Outline the treatment programme for this patient, stressing the nursing involvement.

NURSING THE ANXIOUS PATIENT

Self-Evaluation Test

1. Mr J. has been monopolising the bathroom each morning and missing breakfast, because of his elaborate washing ritual.

Select the best approach to this problem from the list below:

a. insist that he leaves the bathroom and then lock the door;
b. carry out his hygiene for him;
c. allow him to carry out his rituals to their conclusion;
d. suggest to him that he tries to limit his ritual and provide the support and encouragement to help him reach that target.

2. Patients suffering from anxiety states often imagine they have heart diease. This is because . . .

Select the best response from the list below:

a. heart disease is common in chronically anxious people;
b. anxious people often experience angina;
c. they arouse the attention and concern of others in this way;
d. palpitations and chest pain common in anxiety can easily be misinterpreted.

3. Mrs D. has been unable to leave her house without feeling on edge and apprehensive for years. She knows her anxiety is quite irrational, but is unable to control it.

This is an example of . . .

Select the best response from the list below:

a. hypochondriasis;
b. delusions of persecution;
c. obsessional ritual;
d. phobic anxiety.

4. Select from the list below the statement that best describes the technique called 'modelling', used in the treatment of phobic states:

a. the therapist tries to uncover the origins of the phobia;
b. the therapist encourages the patients to imagine themselves in the situation they find distressing and tries to promote a relaxed state;
c. the therapist participates comfortably and confidently in the situation that is causing anxiety while the patient observes;
d. the therapist exposes the patient to the situation that causes maximum anxiety until anxiety begins to diminish.

5. Mr Y. is quite unable to remember who he is, where he lives or any personal details about his life. Despite physical examination no cause can be found for his amnesia.

This is an example of . . .
Select the best response from the list below:

a. Munchausens syndrome;
b. dementia;
c. concussion;
d. conversion reaction.

6. Select from the list below those items which describe the physiological features of anxiety:

a. heart-rate increases;
b. pupils dilate;
c. sweating;
d. blood pressure falls;
e. urge to micturate;
f. muscle tone increases;
g. respiratory rate increases;
h. diarrhoea
(i) a,c,d,e
(ii) a,b,c,e,f,g,h
(iii) a,c,e,f,h
(iv) all of the above.

7. You observe Mrs D. sitting in a corner of the dayroom looking very distracted, tense and anxious.
Select the best approach from the list below:
a. would you like the Doctor to give you something to help you relax, Mrs D.?
b. you seem worried about something this morning, Mrs D. Would it help to talk to me about it?
c. why don't you go and lie on your bed and try to relax?
d. I will take you to the O/T department, Mrs D, it will help keep your mind occupied.

8. What is considered to be the *most* important cause of anorexia nervosa:
a. virus;
b. endocrine disorder;
c. adolescent adjustment difficulties;
d. depression;
e. early weaning from breast/bottle?

9. The physiological changes associated with anxiety are brought about by the . . .

Select the most appropriate response from the list below:

a. central nervous system;
b. thyroid gland;
c. automatic nervous system;
d. pituitary gland.

10. Mrs Chase has been very tense, restless and preoccupied all day. Which of the following activities would be *most* helpful for her:

a. playing a board game;
b. going for a walk with the nurse;
c. participating in a quiz;
d. reading a book?

Assertion and reason

Each of the questions in this section consists of an assertion followed by a reason. Assign to each question one of the five categories (a–e) given in the key below:

KEY

a. The assertion and reason are both true.
The reason is a correct explanation of the assertion.
b. The assertion and reason are both true.
The reason is *not* a correct explanation of the assertion.
c. The assertion is true but the reason is false.
d. The assertion is false but the reason is true.
e. The assertion and reason are both false.

ASSERTION

1. It is important not to respond with too much care and attention to attention-seeking behaviour.

REASON

Attention-seeking would be reinforced.

ASSERTION

2. A 'relationship gap' often opens up between staff and attention-seeking patients.

REASON
People with hysterical personalities find it difficult to sustain relationships.

ASSERTION
3. Behaving in an obsessional way helps reduce anxiety.

REASON
The individual is able to exert maximum control over the events of his life.

ASSERTION
4. Obsessional ruminations often take the form of ideas of a repugnant nature.

REASON
Such ideas express unconscious wishes.

ASSERTION
5. The anorexic patient often shows great interest in buying and preparing food.

REASON
It distracts the attention of others away from their dieting and allays concern.

ASSERTION
6. Restricting privileges in the early stages of treatment is a useful approach to the management of anorexic patients.

REASON
A complete rest is essential.

ASSERTION
7. The use of negative reinforcement in the behavioural management of attention-seekers is often unhelpful.

REASON
It increases insecurity and anxiety and precipitates further attention-seeking.

ASSERTION
8. A feature of tension headaches is nausea and vomiting.

REASON
Aspirin irritates the mucosa of the stomach.

ASSERTION
9. The modern nuclear family is a more stable unit emotionally than the extended family.

REASON
Couples have to rely on each other more for support and satisfaction.

ASSERTION
10. Some anxious, frustrated people get a sense of security from overeating.

REASON
In infancy anxieties are calmed by the bottle or breast, this source of comfort is never completely abandoned.

True/False Items

1. Extreme weight loss, loss of appetite, menorrhagia, and denial are all features of anorexia nervosa. (True; False)
2. People who behave in attention-seeking ways are always conscious of their motives. (True; False)
3. Anxiety should be regarded as a normal and desirable human characteristic. (True; False).
4. Biofeedback is a special diet used for treating some psychosomatic illness. (True; False)
5. Anxiety may inhibit sexual performance. (True; False)
6. Pain may be tolerated more easily if it is anticipated and understood by the patient. (True; False)
7. The enthusiasm and interest of the staff often contributes as much in successful treatment as the treatment itself. (True; False)
8. Many of the frustrations of early marriage arise because idealised expectations are not achieved. (True; False)
9. In phobic anxiety generalisation of the fear stimulus means the person becomes very anxious about life in general. (True; False)
10. An elderly bereaved man is more likely to become socially isolated than a bereaved woman. (True; False)

REFERENCES AND FURTHER READING

Bowlby, J. (1975), *Separation*, Pelican.
Dominian, J. (1968), *Marital Breakdown*, Pelican.
Fletcher, R. (1974), *The Marriage and Family in Britain*, Pelican.
Gillis, L. (1978), *Human Behaviour in Illness*, Faber.
Hilgard, R., Atkinson, R. C., and Atkinson, R. L. (1975), *Introduction to Psychology*, 6th edition, Harcourt Brace Jovanovich.
Mereness, D. (1978), *Essentials of Psychiatric Nursing*, Mosby.
Mitchell, R. (1974), *Advances in Psychiatry*, 'Nursing Times' Publications.
Rachman, S. J. (1978), *Psychology of Medicine*, Pelican.
Rycroft, C. (1970), *Anxiety and Neurosis*, Pelican.
Seyle, H. (1956), *The Stress of Life*, McGraw-Hill.
Wilson-Barnett, J. (1976), Patients emotional reactions to hospitalisation, *Journal of Advanced Nursing*, **1**, 5.
Wolf, H., Wolf, G. (1950), *Life Stress and Disease*, Williams & Wilkins.

Unit 5

The Problem of Aggression

INTRODUCTION

At one time aggressive, violent behaviour was an everyday occurrence in mental hospitals, but with the development of pharmacological treatment during the 1950s, social therapy and the expansion of the open-door policy such behaviour is now relatively infrequent. The open-door policy and the more permissive treatment régimes have, however, made the skilled anticipation of violent behaviour of paramount importance. The current sensitivity of the public, press and health authorities to any hint of 'abuse', coupled with the lack of clear legislative and local guidelines has made the job of ward staff in controlling the violent patient very difficult.

In recent years there has been a steady increase in the incidence of violent crime, domestic violence and violence in the general hospital setting. Many nurses working in the community or in Accident and Emergency departments are faced with the problem of the aggressive drunk or the confused violent patient. The skilled anticipation, prevention, management and evaluation of aggressive episodes are therefore essential parts of the nurse's repertoire of skills.

This unit aims to increase your understanding of the nature of aggression and its relationship with health problems, and to develop your skills in the management of aggressive incidents. (The material contained in this unit on the management of violent incidents is offered as a guide only. Nurses should familiarise themselves with local policy.)

That man is naturally aggressive is a theory that has long been examined by students of human behaviour. The idea that man has an innate aggressive drive or instinct that needs some form of direct or indirect expression is a popular one amongst some psychologists. Much controversy surrounds the possible existence of such an instinct and the part it might play in influencing human behaviour.

There can be no denying that man, like all other animals, has an inbuilt physiological mechanism for expressing the aggressive response. It is obvious that such a mechanism needs to exist to enable an animal to counter possible threats from the environment. What is in doubt is whether there is an internal stimulus for such a response as well as an external one.

1. Define an instinct.

2. Discuss with your group the statement that 'man has an internal need to express aggression, either directly or indirectly'.

If one assumes that such an internal 'trigger mechanism' exists then there are many implications for the nurse. If a natural direct or indirect expression of aggression is denied to the patient over a long period, then the consequences might be either a spontaneous 'explosion' of overt aggression, or an exhibition of self-destructive behaviour (imploded). In some primitive societies a more direct expression of aggression may be acceptable, but in all advanced societies it is actively suppressed. Such suppression has meant that acceptable alternative outlets must be available to allow indirect expression.

The mental mechanism of displacement, discussed in the earlier unit on 'Mental Health', is one way in which aggressive feelings can be ventilated, indirectly. This involves the transfer of the aggressive feelings from the original unacceptable 'target' towards an acceptable substitute.

3. What outlets for aggressive feelings can you suggest from the following patients.

a. The young patient on a short-stay unit
b. A middle-aged patient on a long-stay unit
c. A patient confined to bed or wheelchair.

Alternatively the mechanism of identification may be utilised and the potential aggressor may identify with an aggressive 'hero' figure, and the unacceptable acts and conquests of the hero figure.

Another way of viewing aggression is to see it as being a learned response, and therefore, in an ideal world one that could be completely avoidable. This theory is, of course, directly opposite to the idea of an aggressive instinct.

Whether or not aggression is a response to an external or an internal stimulus, a factor that must be considered is the extent to which an individual is able to control aggression. That a world could be achieved in which aggression no longer exists is obviously unrealistic at present. Nevertheless, it should be possible to reduce the incidence of aggression by demonstrating more healthy ways of dealing with stress and frustration, other than a violent reaction to it.

The concept of role models and their importance in emotional development was also discussed in the unit on 'Mental Health'. The different ways that young children see potentially aggressive situations resolved by their parents and other important role figures must obviously influence the ways they handle such situations. Again they will identify with their parents, and also perhaps with heroes from the popular television programmes and films, and they may try out what they have learned in play situations with their play group. At the same time social learning processes should encourage the development of a guilt response to anti-social behaviour, and the development of a conscience should act as a deterrent to aggression.

Aggression that is controlled may well be a desirable characteristic as it can be an important drive or 'energy source' for much constructive behaviour. A complete lack of aggression may be as serious an indication of personality disorder as too much aggression.

Nurses in hospitals are dealing mainly with adults whose behaviour patterns are well established. Nevertheless by acting as a role model for patients, the nurse is often able to demonstrate a well-balanced attitude towards frustrating and threatening situations that can occur on the ward.

4. Consider what type of patients you have nursed/are nursing that would most benefit from such role modelling.

Most nurses in psychiatric hospitals, on occasions, have to restrain patients who are being aggressive.

5. Discuss with your group how the nurse can avoid or reduce losing credibility as a role model when dealing with such situations.

There is yet a third theory to the origin of aggression and that is, whether it be innate or learned, it occurs only as a response to frustration. This hypothesis assumes that when an individual's efforts to reach a goal are thwarted, this will often stimulate an aggressive drive; this in turn, will motivate aggressive behaviour towards the cause of the frustration. Thus, aggression may not be inborn, but in a world such as ours frustration is inevitable, and so an aggressive drive is an almost universal state.

Refer to Unit 1 on 'Mental Health' and to the hierarchy of individual needs as seen by Maslow. There are obviously many potential barriers to the satisfaction of these needs, and therefore many causes of frustration.

It should be clear from this that one way of reducing the incidence of aggression would be to reduce causes of frustration. Obviously this is a very difficult task, but, nevertheless, there are probably many situations that commonly cause frustrations for patients both inside and outside the hospital that could be improved.

6. Identify at least three common causes of frustration for patients in the following situations:

a. A short-stay admission unit
b. A Casualty or Outpatients department
c. A long-stay ward.

7. How easy would it be to reduce or remove the frustrating situations you have mentioned?

The theories may show the possible origins of aggressive behaviour but a knowledge of them will not, in themselves, prepare the nurse effectively to deal with a violent incident. Their value lies in indicating possible short- and long-term measures.

Aggressive incidents occur for many apparent reasons, although some psychologists distinguish between two basic types of motivation for aggressive behaviour.

i. *Hostile aggression*, the aim of which is to inflict injury.
ii. *Instrumental aggression*, which is aimed at a goal other than the victim's injury; that is, it is a means to an end.

It is not always clear which is which, and the nurse will see both types of aggression. Neither is easy to manage but the latter is likely to be more of a long-term problem.

Violence in Casualty departments has long been a problem and is currently on the increase. Dealing with drunks on a Saturday night has always contained the threat of violence, but the increasing tendency for other types of patient to attack nurses and doctors is growing cause for concern.

Equally, violence towards babies, children and towards wives has received much publicity in recent years. It may be that it is an increasing problem, or that as a society we are more aware of it and the need to do something about it. Either way, non-accidental injury of children is difficult to understand, particularly for many people who have not experienced the trials and tribulations of parenthood, and often for those who have. Any of the explanations of aggression mentioned earlier could explain why it happens; yet it is difficult for many to sympathise with persons with a history of violence towards children. The nurse must be as objective as possible about such patients and in their assessment of the causes of the situation and evaluation of the patient's needs.

8. Using your knowledge of the causes of aggression, write a descriptive profile of:

a. A woman who is likely to batter her baby
b. A man who is likely to batter his wife.

Many Health Authorities prepare checklists of factors which, if present, point to a possibility of actual or potential physical abuse towards children. Perhaps only one or two may be present but the presence of any should alert health workers, particularly Community Nurses, Health Visitors and staff in Casualty departments, to carry out a thorough assessment.

Below are given some points that would be on such a checklist.

9. Complete the list for both the parent and the child.

THE PARENT

a. Consistently complains of the child being bad, difficult to manage or 'different' from other children
b. Relates a history of rejection or abuse in own childhood
c. Shows inappropriate attachment when child has been injured
d. Has a psychopathic personality.
e.
f.
g.
h.

THE CHILD

a. Appears unnaturally concerned about parents' needs

b. Shows evidence of repeated skin injuries. Injuries specially to note are:

(i) bruising to head or cheek
(ii) bites.
(iii)
(iv)

c.
d.
e.

10. Steve and Jane S., both aged 22, have been married two years and have a daughter Sarah aged ten months. They live in a small flat on the top floor of a large house in an area of town that is in social decline. They have been saving hard for a home of their own, but then Jane became pregnant and had to give up work. Since then they have been able to save very little. Steve is a bus driver and works a great deal of overtime.

Jane is an only child of middle-class parents. She was very lonely as a child and was left alone a lot by her parents who were too preoccupied with their own careers and interests to give her much attention. Steve was her first serious boy-friend and was rather 'bulldozed' into an early marriage by Jane. Jane's parents disapproved of Steve and now have only occasional contact with her.

Jane had an uncomfortable pregnancy and Sarah was born four weeks prematurely. She had no real experience of young babies and during the early weeks felt very clumsy and inadequate with Sarah. Initially Jane felt very loving towards the child and was determined to give the child the warm, caring mothering she had missed. Sarah was not an easy child to nurse – she was fretful, difficult with feeds and often had long crying spells at night. Jane could never seem to satisfy her and began to feel Sarah was rejecting her. As the months went by Jane felt more and more that Sarah was being deliberately wilful in such things as soiling, refusing her feed, wriggling and kicking when she tried to dress her; also Sarah would often pull away when Jane tried to cuddle her.

Over the past two to three months Jane has become depressed, and apathetic and indifferent towards Sarah. She has begun to feed her irregularly and in moments of frustration and anger – usually triggered by a row with Steve or the baby soiling or crying, has violently shaken, slapped or thrown Sarah about.

Steve is a rather demanding, self-centred person who was 'spoilt' by his doting, capable mother. Steve tends to get angry if things don't go his way. He works hard at his job and is frustrated by their lack of social progress. He enjoys a pint and plays sport at the weekends. He is not very supportive towards Jane and thinks she should be able to cope. He expects her time and attention when he gets home at night and gets angry if the baby interferes.

Suspicions are aroused when Jane takes Sarah to the local clinic. Bruising is noticed for which Jane cannot give an adequate explanation and the child is clearly underweight. She is also unusually stiff and passive and watchful when handled. Jane's GP and health visitor are alerted.

i. Mother Burns Baby With a Cigarette', 'Father Punches Three-Year-Old Son Fracturing His Jaw', 'Two-Year-Old Girl Starved to Death by Her Parents'. These are sadly common headlines in the popular press. Examine your attitudes towards such people.
ii. Identify the factors which may have contributed to abuse in the case of Sarah.
iii. Outline the ways in which this family could be helped.

It is unfortunately true that aggressive behaviour has always been associated with psychiatric hospitals. In the minds of many people, therefore, violence has been regarded as an inevitable and integral symptom of psychiatric illness. This is not generally so; violence is not a primary symptom of any illness but is a secondary result of some. The possible exception is the psychopathic patient, in whom aggression is often the central feature and persistently disrupts the individual's social functioning and threatens the well-being of others.

Man's ability to cope with his environment effectively depends to a large extent on his ability to perceive reality correctly and understand it. Anything that interferes with the individual's perception of reality – either by blocking it or distorting it, or interfering with their understanding of it, obviously increases the risk of that individual feeling threatened. For that reason certain types of psychiatric illness are more likely to have aggressive responses as a feature than others.

Any patient who is confused and disorientated may become aggressive in some circumstances. Such patients are not normally aggressive, but when confused their inability to understand their environment, and the increased likelihood of their misinterpreting it, frequently results in aggressive resistive behaviour. This is just as likely to happen in general hospitals as in psychiatric hospitals. The risk is increased if the patients' hearing or sight is impaired, for example in the elderly.

11. Determine in which physical and psychiatric states confusion is likely to diminish the patient's grasp on reality and possibly result in aggressive behaviour.

In the psychiatric hospital the two most obvious ways in which reality is distorted is by delusions and hallucinations.

12. Discuss specific ways in which the following could stimulate aggressive behaviour:

a. Paranoid delusions
b. Grandiose delusions.

There are many ways in which hallucinations can stimulate aggression. A good example is in alcoholism during the stage of alcohol withdrawal. Hallucinations occur frequently, particularly frightening visual and tactile hallucinations. The patient will often attack the nursing staff, who may well appear grossly distorted.

(Refer to Unit 7 on 'Alcohol/Drug Dependence').

13. Consider other specific ways in which hallucinations can cause aggression.

The type of aggression that occurs in confusional states and psychotic conditions is usually of the *hostile* variety, and the long-term management of this problem usually revolves round relief of the underlying condition causing the confusion, or alleviation of the psychotic state. This usually removes the threat of aggressive behaviour.

Instrumental aggression, in which the patient uses the threat or act of violence as a manipulative device, can be an even bigger problem in psychiatric hospitals. Such violence is often directed toward windows or furniture rather than staff, and as such can often be regarded as an attempt to achieve some end.

Alternatively it may be an expression of frustration by the patient and the displaced source may not be easily recognisable.

When managing aggression that is essentially manipulative, a consistent, patient and flexible approach by the treatment team is obviously vital. The aim must be to help the patient learn that aggressive manipulation causes more problems than it solves, and that a modification of their behaviour will bring its own reward in terms of more permanently improved interpersonal relationships. The success that has been achieved with this type of patient has been largely gained through the group approach, rather than through an individual psychotherapeutic one. Such patients appear to respond best to treatment in a therapeutic community setting.

Individual members are consistently confronted with the results of their anti-social actions by the other group members and may, as a result of this coercive group pressure, be forced to modify their behaviour in order to avoid rejection from the group. Hopefully, the rewards gained from such a change in behaviour will increase the individual's insight into the shortcomings of his previous behaviour, and will act as a spur in making his improved behaviour a more permanent state.

It may well be that certain aspects of the hospital 'milieu' can act as 'trigger' factors for aggressive behaviour.

Certainly a stay in hospital under the compulsory admission and detention orders of the 1959 Mental Health Act could well lead to violent response. There are, of necessity, a small group of patients in psychiatric hospitals whose mental state requires that they be detained against their will. Their hold on reality is frequently impaired, and this, coupled with their loss of freedom, can obviously result in aggressive reactions. There is little the nurses can do to prevent this situation arising. Their main aim must be to ensure that any aggressive episodes are resolved correctly, that the patient retains as much dignity and independence as possible, and the treatment team must see that any restrictions that are imposed should last only as long as the patient's mental state dictates.

14. Describe how the following factors might stimulate aggression. In each case consider what should be done to avoid/reduce their effects:

a. Attitudes of the staff
b. Overcrowding
c. Boredom
d. Personality clashes
e. Jealousy
f. Medication administration
g. Visiting times
h. Sexual restrictions.

MANAGEMENT OF AGGRESSIVE EPISODES

Even in the best-run wards/units, despite vigorous efforts to reduce the likelihood of violent incidents, there will be occasions when threatened or actual violence will take place. The correct management and resolution of these situations is obviously of paramount importance.

It is essential for nurses to be aware of their own reactions to aggressive situations as reactions influence the way in which situations are dealt with. Obviously the nurse who reacts to violence with violence will only serve to inflame the situation further.

15. Identify with your group other undesirable reactions to violence. What can be done to improve them?

When coping with both threatened and actual violence, a comprehensive knowledge of the patient and a sound nurse–patient relationship are obvious advantages.

If it becomes apparent that the patient is likely to become violent, then the nurse should do nothing that is likely to be mistaken for aggression on her part. She should talk quietly to the patient and try to relieve the tension in an effort to 'defuse' the situation. Very often feelings are infectious and the calm, relaxed mood of the nurses (which may take a great effort to maintain) can be transmitted to the patient and avert the aggressive incident. It may be possible to determine the source of the patient's anxiety or frustration and provide the necessary reassurance or take some immediate action to reduce the patient's sense of frustration.

The senior nurse on the ward should ensure that there are sufficient staff to deal with the incident. It may be that a show of force, albeit intimidatory, may deter the patient from his aggressive aim.

In the event of violent behaviour occurring it may be appropriate to give prescribed medication. This may prevent a serious incident but sometimes may itself precipitate further violence. The senior nurse must use her judgement to decide if the risk should be taken. If it is decided that the administration of drugs is essential, then the patient should be approached calmly by the nurse and the drug offered. If the patient refuses to take them, despite the nurses efforts to persuade otherwise, then the medical officer responsible should be informed in order to decide whether the drugs should be given against the patient's wishes.

16. Discuss with your group what situations might merit the administration of drugs against the patient's wishes.

If violence occurs then it should be treated like any other emergency. Assistance should be sought using whatever emergency call system is appropriate. Medical and senior nursing staff should attend at once.

It is essential that priority be given to the protection of other patients and staff, and damage to property is of secondary importance unless of course the patient is likely to injure himself seriously. If a member of the staff is alone, he is entitled to take whatever steps are appropriate to protect himself from injury.

If there is time, it is a wise precaution for nurses to remove objects that might be broken or that might injure either nurse or patient (for example, pens, watches, spectacles) before restraining the patient.

Whilst restraining the patient pressure should never be put on the patient's head, throat, chest or abdomen; this can cause serious injury. If it is possible the patient should be restrained by his clothes, rather than his limbs.

There should be enough staff present to immobilise the patient quickly, and this is best done against a wall, or better still, on the floor. Restraint can be continued by the nurses holding the patient firmly by the shoulders and arms, pelvis and legs. The patient's shoes should be removed whenever possible. Throughout the period of restraint the nurse must continue to talk to the patient in an effort to calm and reassure him/her.

The patient must never be struck, either by hand or by any other weapon, and the amount of force used should be the minimum required to restrain the patient safely and control the situation.

Medication may be given if necessary, and the patient should be removed to a seclusion room if disturbed aggressive behaviour seems likely to continue. Staff should stay with the patient until the drug begins to take effect and the patient becomes more controlled and composed. Other patients should be reassured and calmed following the incident.

17. Aggression often appears to be 'contagious', and the aggressive incident may be followed by seemingly unconnected further incidents involving other patients. Why may this be so?

It is essential that the incident be reported fully, both clinically and administratively, using Incident Report forms and Accident Report forms if necessary.

Violence is undignified both for the nurses and for the patient, and as soon as possible after the incident dignity must be restored. How this is done depends largely on the nurses' attitude towards the patient. If it is transmitted to the patient that nurses both fear and resent him/her, this is likely to lead to further violence. It is vital to show the patient that the incident has not harmed the nurses' relationship with him/her. The nurse must be allowed to show disappointment and disapproval if this is indicated, but not condemnation. This is particularly important if the patient is secluded following the incident. The period of seclusion must be as short as possible and only be used for the protection of the patient or others; never as a punishment. During the period of seclusion strict observation must be maintained because the patient, possibly motivated by remorse, may resort to self-destructive behaviour. Attention to diet, hygiene and toileting needs should be carefully maintained. As soon as possible after the incident, the treatment team and the patient must meet to discuss the causes of the incident and what should be done to prevent its reoccurrence.

Ward/unit community meetings will also need to consider the effects of the incident, and the nurses must help the community understand the patient's violence, and to understand the staff's handling of it.

The treatment team should meet separately to discuss its management of the situation. For all concerned the incident must be kept in proportion, and if it is used as a learning situation, some benefit might be derived from it.

One of the most frightening, and fortunately infrequent, situations of violence is that in which a patient has a dangerous weapon such as a knife or even a firearm. In these situations the nurse must err absolutely on the side of caution and display no heroics. Unless actually attacked the nurses should do nothing to disarm or antagonise the patient, but should remove as many persons as possible who are at risk and contact the police immediately. They are trained to deal with such situations far more effectively than nurses. The nurses should do all that is demanded of them by the patient, other than putting persons further at risk, until the police arrive.

For nurses working in the community the threat of violence poses different problems. The patient is at home; members of the patient's family may be present and the nurse is quite likely to be alone. If the patient does threaten violence then the nurse should use the same skills of counselling and persuasion that would be used in the hospital situation, in an attempt to calm the patient.

If an attack takes place in the patient's home then the nurse must obviously defend herself and if restraint and control are unlikely to be achieved she should leave the situation and report to her senior colleagues. Because the nurse is likely to be isolated in this situation more than any other, prevention based on skilled anticipation is essential. If the nurse is in any doubt before entering the patient's home she should seek assistance before going in. If when a home visit is being planned the nurse anticipates that the patient might become aggressive then it would be wise to visit with a colleague.

18. Select a patient you have nursed who has behaved in an aggressive/violent way. Identify the reasons for his/her behaviour.

19. Discuss the way in which the incident was controlled and how further similar incidents were/could be prevented.

20. You are visiting Mr Arthur D., aged 71, in his home. Mr D. suffers from dementia and has regular spells in and out of hospital. While he is at home he is supported by the community nurse who visits twice a week. On this occasion he appears very confused and has been quite aggressive towards his wife who is very distressed as a result. He obviously does not recognise you on your arrival and accuses you of trying to steal his life savings. Mr D. becomes very excitable and aggressive and lashes out at you.

Try and imagine yourself in this situation. Discuss the ways in which you might best resolve it.

21. Mrs Cristabell N., aged 34, is a patient on your ward being treated for hypomania. She is detained in hospital under Section 25 of the Mental Health Act. At the moment she is very restless and garrulous; at times she is elated, excitable and grandiose. There is clearly a need to maintain a quiet, calm environment at this time. It is Sunday morning and Cristabell wants to go to church. This is clearly not advisable but she will not be persuaded and attempts aggressively to push past you and leave the ward.

Try and imagine yourself in this situation. Discuss the ways in which you might best resolve it.

THE AGGRESSIVE PATIENT

Self-Evaluation Test

Choose the most suitable answer from the four given:

1. In psychological terms the word instinctive means:

a. a learned response that is unconscious;

b. an inborn tendency to react in a definite pattern of behaviour;
c. a particular type of awareness or 'sixth sense';
d. uncontrollable urges or compulsions that direct all our behaviour.

2. The redirection of aggression from an unacceptable target towards a more acceptable substitute object is:

a. transference;
b. sublimation;
c. delegation;
d. displacement

3. If a patient appears to threaten aggression, the nurse should always:

a. try to remain as calm and unruffled as possible;
b. shout loudly for assistance from colleagues;
c. attempt to trap the patient against a wall;
d. ignore the patient and pretend to have noticed nothing.

4. Some aggressive incidents may be prevented by nurses who have a sound knowledge of individual patients. This is because:

a. the nurse will know a patient's weaknesses and how to use them;
b. the nurse will be able to anticipate many situations that may threaten violence;
c. the nurse will have something in common with the patient to talk about;
d. the nurse will be able to report objectively about the patient after any violent episode.

5. Following aggressive incidents, long periods of seclusion should be avoided whenever possible. This is because:

a. it is illegal to seclude patients for more than four hours without medical direction;
b. patients are frequently a fire hazard whilst nursed in seclusion;
c. there is a likelihood of the patient feeling punished and rejected during seclusion;
d. long periods of seclusion frequently result in a poor standard of diet and hygiene for the patient.

6. It is not uncommon for one aggressive incident to be followed by another involving other patients. This is most often caused by:

a. an increase in tension and insecurity on the ward following the first incident;
b. patients looking for revenge against the nurses for their handling of the first incident;
c. the nurses are often irritable and short-tempered following an aggressive incident;
d. patients often feel that they should 'finish off' the aggressive behaviour started by the other patients.

7. During the actual management of an aggressive incident, at least one nurse should be available to care for those patients not involved, whenever the situation allows. This is because:

a. there is a danger that they will rush to help the aggressive patient;
b. it is likely that patients will be required to carry messages to help resolve the incident;
c. the nurse will be able to explain to the other patients exactly what caused the incident;
d. most patients find aggressive incidents extremely disturbing and distressing and require reassurance.

Assertion and reason

Each of the questions in this section consists of an assertion followed by a reason. Assign to each question one of the five categories (a–e) given in the key below:

KEY

a. The assertion and reason are both true.
The reason is a correct explanation of the assertion.
b. The assertion and reason are both true.
The reason is *not* a correct explanation of the assertion.
c. The assertion is true but the reason is false.
d. The assertion is false but the reason is true.
e. The assertion and reason are both false.

ASSERTION
1. Skilful observation of a patient's general behaviour plays an important part in preventing aggression.

REASON
If patients appreciate they are being observed they will behave themselves.

ASSERTION

2. It is essential to allow patients as much personal freedom as possible.

REASON

Suppressive nursing techniques are likely to cause an increase in aggressive incidents.

ASSERTION

3. Aggressive behaviour, when expressed in an acceptable manner, is an essential part of the range of normal human behaviour.

REASON

It is not helpful for nurses to take a punitive attitude toward aggression.

ASSERTION

4. The incidence of aggressive behaviour is less amongst the mentally ill than the general population.

REASON

Some mental illnesses have the effect of lowering drive and motivation.

5. Sufficient staffing levels are essential in preventing aggressive incidents occurring.

REASON

If patients realise that there are many nurses on the ward they will be deterred from starting trouble.

ASSERTION

6. Junior nurses should be supported in their care of patients who are potentially violent.

REASON

Insecurity experienced by nurses may be transmitted to patients, causing them to feel insecure, and possibly aggressive.

ASSERTION

7. As soon as possible after an aggressive incident the events should be discussed at a multidisciplinary staff meeting.

REASON
If there is a delay between aggressive incidents and staff evaluation meetings, reactions to such incidents may become stereotyped and non-therapeutic.

ASSERTION
8. If a community nurse is alone and faced by a violent situation, she should stand firm and resist the patient.

REASON
A community nurse will 'lose face' with the patient if she retreats from violent situations.

True/False items

1. Regular ward meetings will help reduce the incidence of aggression. (True; False)
2. Aggressive feelings can be expressed in ways other than by aggressive behaviour. (True; False)
3. It is important that nurses be physically strong in order to cope with aggression. (True; False)
4. A nurse's general attitudes could be instrumental in stimulating aggressive responses. (True; False)
5. Nurses must learn not to feel fear and anxiety when confronted by aggressive behaviour. (True; False)
6. Most battered wives are women who married young and impulsively. (True; False)
7. Wife battering is more common amongst the immigrant population than amongst the indigenous population of the U.K. (True; False)
8. Aggression is a prominent symptom of most psychotic illnesses. (True; False)
9. Mentally handicapped people are more likely to be aggressive than people of normal intelligence. (True; False)
10. Many parents who physically abuse children were themselves abused by their own parents. (True; False)

REFERENCES AND FURTHER READING

Ardrey, R. (1970), *The Social Contract*, Collins.
Burgess, A. (1972), *A Clockwork Orange*, Penguin.

Chalmers, N., Crawley, R., and Rose, S. (1975), *The Biological Bases of Behaviour*, Harper & Row.
Hilgard, R., Atkinson, R. C., and Atkinson, R. L. (1975), *Introduction to Psychology*, 6th edition, Harcourt Brace Jovanovich.
Howells, J. G. (1974), *Remember Maria*, Butterworths.
Mark, Sir Robert (1977), *Policing a Perplexed Society*, George Allen & Unwin.
Mitchell, Dr A. R. K. (1978), *Violence in the Family*, Wayland.
Pizzey, E. (1978), *Infernal Child*, Victor Gollancz.
Storr, A. (1968), *Human Aggression*, Penguin.
Toch, H. (1972), *Violent Men*, Penguin/Pelican.

Unit 6

Nursing the Confused Patient

INTRODUCTION

We use the term 'confusion' in everyday language to describe our reactions to information and events we are unable to understand. Our inability to comprehend may be because there is too much to take in; the information is too difficult; poorly presented, or because it is totally unfamiliar to us. The term is also widely used medically to describe the behaviour of people who, because their brain function has deteriorated, are unable to comprehend and respond rationally to their environments. It is usual to describe these disorders of brain function in two main groups. First the acute confusional states (delirium) which are of sudden onset and result in temporary confusion; and secondly the chronic confusional states (dementia) in which the disability is of a more progressive and permanent nature. Pathological confusion can occur at any age, but it is most commonly encountered in the elderly who are very vulnerable to the dementias and to the cerebral effects of various medical disorders.

We live in an ageing population. Advances in medical technology and improvements in living standards have increased the number of people surviving into their seventh and eighth decades from 3 to 6 million. But while the impact of medical science on those diseases such as tuberculosis and diphtheria has made longevity an expectation rather than a bonus, it has had little impact on the degenerative diseases that affect people in the latter years of their lives. With more people surviving to suffer from these diseases a great strain has been put on the health care resources in the United Kingdom. The psychiatric services are particularly affected and currently around 50 per cent of the in-patient population are over 65 and in addition an increasing number of elderly people are being supported by expanding community services.

This unit is therefore mainly concerned with the care of the elderly patient, but much of the discussion is relevant to the care of confused patients of all ages. The aim of this unit is to increase your background knowledge of the principal disorders which result in confused behaviour, and to develop your skills in the management of such patients.

Senile dementia is a common cause of confused behaviour affecting elderly people in their 70s and 80s. More women than men are affected. For some reason yet unknown there is a rapid and progressive degeneration of the cortical neurones, resulting in brain atrophy and a progressive deterioration in mental ability and social behaviour.

The onset is gradual; the early signs being muddled, forgetful, careless behaviour. Things are mislaid, names forgotten and familiar tasks become increasingly difficult. The individual often tries to cover up for these disabilities by making excuses, laughing them off, or restricting his life style. Hygiene, diet and dress may be neglected and, as the disorder progresses, memory, particularly for recent events) becomes very patchy. Memory gaps may be filled with confabulations. Disorientation for time, place and person becomes prominent, so that the patient may mistake the nurse for his wife or daughter and the ward day-room for his own living-room. The ability to make sense of his surroundings and cope with everyday activities is gradually lost, often with understandable perplexity and anxiety. Coherent speech becomes replaced by fragmented, muddled conversation. Sometimes patients become apathetic and withdrawn, showing little interest in their environments, while others may be restless and labile in mood. Insomnia and nocturnal confusion may be a problem.

Aggressive paranoid outbursts occur from time to time and are usually related to the misinterpretation of events. Some personal possession may have been mislaid and a staff member or fellow patient accused of taking it, or staff may be accused by a patient of molesting them as they assist them with dressing or hygiene. Previous personality traits and sometimes anti-social behaviour may become prominent as inhibition is lost, resulting in mischievous or coarse behaviour; occasionally more serious sexual aberrations occur.

Social behaviour deteriorates as the disorder progresses, the patient requiring support and supervision with washing, feeding and dressing. Incontinence, wandering, and nocturnal confusion may be a problem. In the terminal stages the patient becomes very frail and emaciated, and may have to be nursed in bed requiring a great deal of care to ensure comfort is maintained until death.

It is important that disorders such as senile dementia are recognized in the early stages so that supportive care can be provided and the patient's independence and safety maintained. It is usually possible for patients to be maintained in their own homes for some time, providing appropriate help can be mobilised. Often some concurrent psychiatric, medical or social problem such as depression, a chest infection or the illness of a supportive relative will supervene and exacerbate the patient's problems. If these factors can be identified and resolved there is often a considerable improvement in the patient's behaviour. It is important that nurses are able to recognise the clinical features of depression, which is quite common in old age. Retardation, loss of interest and poor concentration are common characteristics of this illness, and often give a picture of neglect and muddled thinking that can easily be mistaken for dementia.

Thus there is often a firm basis for therapeutic optimism. Much can be done to improve mental clarity and social functioning, and even where deterioration is severe, independence, identity and dignity can be maintained in the simplified and supportive environment of a community home or hospital ward. It is important that nurses should approach the care of such patients with an attitude of expectancy and optimism. The self-fulfilling prophecy is very relevant to the care of the elderly; if people are treated as being incapable and unresponsive, they will become so!

1. The following are also important causes of dementia. Write a concise account of the clinical features of these disorders:

i. Arteriosclerotic dementia
ii. Huntington's chorea
iii. Alzheimer's disease
iv. Alcoholic dementia
v. Cerebral syphilis.

Although what we are describing here is primarily an organic syndrome, it is important to keep in mind the social and psychological experience of the patient which may colour and exacerbate confused behaviour.

As a social group, the elderly are vulnerable to the experience of isolation and loneliness. Man is a social animal; his social and psychological needs are satisfied largely through contact and companionship with others. His behaviour is modified and refined by the influence and expectations of others in the social groups to which he belongs. This is no less true for the elderly and we should therefore not be surprised that eccentricity, anxiety and unhappiness follow in the wake of social isolation.

2. What are the reasons for social isolation in old age?

3. Discuss how you might use your contact with confused patients to meet their need for secuirty, esteem, love and belonging.

4. Occupational disengagement should not result in social disengagement and inactivity if mental health is to be preserved. Consider how this might be avoided.

Man has a nervous system that requires an optimum level of stimulus in order to maintain healthy functioning. Numerous studies have shown that where sensory input is significantly reduced, thought processes, perceptual ability and affective responses become less efficient. Muddled thinking often occurs, bizarre ideas may be expressed, disorientation develops, day-dreaming increases, hallucinations and illusions may be experienced. Mood often becomes depressed or anxious, and the individual may become inert and apathetic. The elderly, because of mobility problems, social isolation, failing vision or hearing, may have a very restricted sensory experience.

5. Discuss the implications of sensory deprivation for the care of the elderly confused patient, both in the community and in hospital.

We have seen that disorientation is a common feature of the dementias and a facet of confused behaviour. Disorientation may be the result of a lack of information rather than a failure to comprehend or memory dysfunction. If a patient has not been told clearly where she is, or has not seen a calendar for some time, then understandably she will be 'disorientated'. Disorientation may also be related to a denial of the unpleasant reality of her circumstances; mistaking the ward day-room for her own sitting-room or the doctor for her husband may be an example of this.

6. Mrs Kate G., aged 73, suffers from dementia and she has been in hospital for four months; she was admitted following the death of her husband who cared for her at home. Kate is moderately confused, at times incontinent, and needs supervision with her dress and hygiene. She has difficulty finding her way round the ward and is frequently found looking lost and bemused. Kate tends to live in the past and frequently says things like 'I must go and get tea ready for Alf' [her husband], and often mistakes the nurses for her daughter. When asked about the time of day or year Kate is usually hopelessly wrong.

i. How may the ward environment be geared to help reduce disorientation?
ii. How could the nurses use their contact with Mrs G. to improve orientation?

We have already commented on how aggressive paranoid behaviour may occur in dementia usually as the result of memory dysfunction and misinterpretation of events. Such outbursts are usually of short duration and the nurse should intervene to protect others and in order to maintain the dignity of the patient. She should try and be calm and reassuring and as the patient becomes more composed and receptive she should try and explain events to the patient. He may mistake his medication for poison, or mistake clothes other patients are wearing for his own, but such notions can usually be dissipated by patient and clear explanations. Resistiveness to care without the paranoid element can also be a problem. Again this often arises because of the misinterpretation of events. The patient cannot understand what it is the nurse is trying to do for him and therefore becomes anxious and aggressive. It is very important that nurses take the trouble to explain slowly and simply what it is they want to do before carrying out care. Sometimes resistiveness occurs because the patient feels frustrated and resentful at the loss of independence and dignity that is imposed on him as the result of hospitalisation and illness. Nurses should remember to encourage self-reliance and self-care wherever possible.

7. Mr Brian D., aged 53, suffers from Huntington's chorea; the first symptoms of the illness appeared about five years ago and he is now permanently hospitalised although he is able to spend the occcasional day at home. His choreiform movements make it difficult for him to meet his personal needs unaided, although he can manage to feed, wash and dress himself given time. Conversation is difficult as his speech is impaired. Dysphagia has become more troublesome recently. Brian appears moderately confused but maintains some appreciation of his circumstances. He often becomes upset and is resistive and aggressive towards the staff when they try to help him. At times he appears quite depressed.

   Discuss how you might improve the morale and reduce aggressive behaviour in this patient.

Deterioration of memory is a key feature of confused behaviour. The two-phase theory of memory suggests that information is stored as memory traces in the form of structural or physiological changes in the brain cells. Initially information is held in a short-term memory bank perhaps in the form of electrical impulses. After a variable period of time, it is consolidated in the more durable long-term memory store in the form of RNA molecules. Information being held in the short-term memory is very vulnerable to disruption and loss, and only a limited amount of information can be held at any one time. Patients suffering from concussion often lose the ability to recall their accidents or events leading up to the accident. Following electro-convulsive therapy patients often cannot remember having treatment. In confusion it is again the short-term memory that is most seriously affected and the patient's capacity to hold and transfer information to the long-term store is extremely reduced.

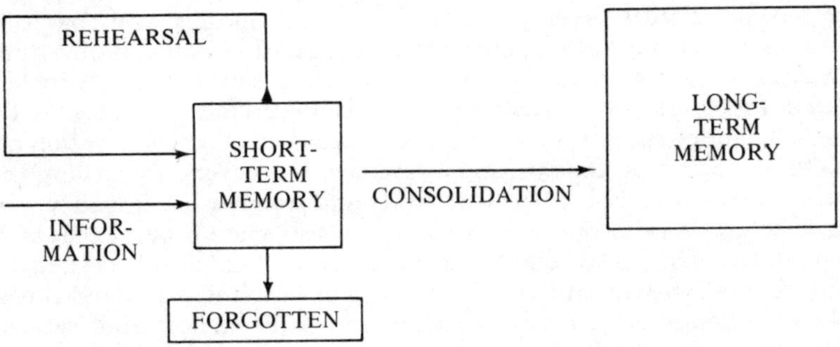

8. The diagram represents the two-phase theory of memory.
  i. Discuss the reasons why people forget
  ii. Identify the factors that help us remember things
  iii. What are the implications for the care of confused patients?

For a person whose mental abilities are failing, being admitted to hospital can prove something of a crisis. Faced with unfamiliar surroundings, unfamiliar people, and a strange new daily routine, their confusion may increase and their behaviour become more disorganized and dependent. It is very important that nurses help the patient settle in properly – explain to he patient where he is – who they are – and what is happening, and show him round the ward. A simple, consistent daily routine should be established as soon as possible in which self-reliance is encouraged where possible and support and supervision given where necessary.

Always sleeping in the same bed, having clothes put out for the morning, being shown to the bathroom, having toiletries set out for you, sitting at the same meal table each day, and having a knife and fork handed to you are examples of supportive elements in the daily routine that can help patients retain some measure of dignity and independence.

9. The individuality and personal identity of elderly patients receiving hospital care is often lost.
Discuss the ways in which this can be prevented.

Activities of an occupational and social nature are very important in the care of the elderly confused patient. Enforced idleness encourages inertia and withdrawal and increases confused thinking. Activities can help promote mental clarity, encourage socialisation and improve mobility. Many activities may be carried out on a group basis; some may be purely recreational, while others have a definite rehabilitative function. Simple craft-work, art, listening to music, music and movement sessions, are all pleasurable and helpful activities; so are simple discussion groups on topics such as personal, local or national events. Being read to; nature rambles; indoor gardening and games such as cards, skittles or ring toss, etc, are useful. Many patients benefit from the opportunity to re-establish domestic skills such as cooking, washing, shopping, etc., and where appropriate this should be part of the activity programme.

10. You have been asked to supervise an activity/resocialisation group of ten male and female, moderately confused patients for a week. Outline a programme you think might be useful.

11. You have been asked to supervise a reality orientation group for six moderately confused and socially withdrawn elderly patients. Outline your programme for the half hour session.

12. Mrs Patricia G. aged 70, suffers from dementia. Her memory is poor and she is quite disorientated, particularly for time and place. Mrs G's speech is very muddled and she has great difficulty coping with simple everyday tasks. The aspect of her behaviour that poses the biggest problem, however, is her restless wandering and if left unsupervised she would wander off the ward and get lost, putting herself at risk.
The problem of restlessness is common in chronic confusional states. Sometimes it seems to be related to he patient's disorientated

state of mind; sometimes to people's need to be active; sometimes to an anxious or excited emotional state.
Discuss the ways in which Mrs G.'s restlessness may be managed.

13. Mr Jake F. is a likeable old man of 70 who lives by himself with the support of meals-on-wheels and a home help in a council flat. The police, who have received complaints from people in the neighbourhood that Jake has been seen in the local park exposing himself to girls on their way home from the nearby school, have asked his doctor to visit him.

This is an example of disinhibition with serious social consequences. Disinhibition in a less extreme form is often seen in dementia.

Give examples of disinhibition you have noticed in your patients. Why does it occur?

14. Urinary incontinence is a disability that is frequently associated with dementia. This is partly because cortical inhibition is lost as the result of brain damage, but may also be attributed to the general effects of confusion and the prevailing mood of the patient. Urinary infection and faecal impaction are also common causes of incontinence in the elderly. It should, therefore, be remembered that the causes of incontinence are variable and that your observations of any characteristic pattern or feature to a patient's incontinence may be a valuable guide to accurate diagnosis and effective management. Observe the frequency of incontinence episodes, he volume passed on each occasion, the circumstances in which the patient was incontinent, any general disability that might prevent normal micturition and the attitudes of the patient towards his/her incontinence.

i. Select a patient on your unit who is incontinent. Describe the ways in which this patient's incontinence problem is managed.
ii. What other aids to the management of incontinence do you know of?
iii. Retraining schedules may lead to a patient regaining continence. Describe a retraining schedule for a patient on your unit, showing how behavioural principles may be applied.
iv. What psychological reactions are likely to occur in patients as a result of this incontinence?
v. How may knowledge of these reactions influence your approach to the care of incontinent patients? Be specific.

15. Select a patient you have nursed suffering from a chronic confusional state and describe their behaviour using the following headings:

Memory/orientation	Mood
Interest	Continence
Speech	Hygiene
Ambulation/manipulative ability	Dietary habits

Describe the nursing care programme for this patient showing how its aim is to reduce any disability you have described above.

Acute confusional states (delirium) are common in the elderly. Any disease process that disrupts the functioning of brain cells may produce confusion of sudden onset. The elderly are particularly vulnerable to the cerebral effects of numerous medical disorders, for example infections, and indeed confusion may be the first indication of the presence of the disease. The natural cell 'fall-out' that occurs as part of ageing, and the degenerative changes associated with dementia, reduce the brain's capacity to cope with disruption.

Acute confusion is characterised by restlessness, apprehension, poor concentration and attention. The patient is disorientated and is unable to make sense of his surroundings. Hallucinations, often of a tactile nature, illusions and persecutory delusions may be present.

16. There are many medical disorders which may produce episodes of acute confusion; drug intoxication and withdrawal have already been mentioned in the unit of drug/alcohol abuse.

Identify other common causes.

The acute confused patient is usually very ill. He needs to rest in bed in a quiet, well-lit room or corner of the ward. Owing to the grossly impaired comprehension, any unnecessary noise and activity will increase confusion and apprehension. In a quiet, well-lit room the patient is more likely to be able to maintain a more rational appreciation of his environment. Nurses should attend to the patient in a calm, unhurried way, explaining to the patient simply and clearly what it is they wish to do for him. While carrying out care the nurse should try to improve orientation and provide reassurance. Touch, the tone of the nurses's voice and her own assurance and competence are more important as reassurers than what is said. Because of the restless agitation that is often present such patients will require close supervision and observation to ensure safety is maintained. Attention to general health and physical comfort is an essential element of care.

17. Mrs Elsie D., a widow aged 72, has been admitted to your unit in an acutely confused state. Her GP was called in by the next-door neighbours who reported that Elsie was wandering round her garden in her underclothes and did not seem to recognise them when they went to her aid. Her doctor found little food in her kitchen and the house was cold and neglected. She was known to have a mild degree of dementia but had been managing well with limited support from social services. Elsie now appears very restless, agitated and confused. She calls out to people, mistaking them for others. Her conversation is often rambling and incoherent and she appears to experience auditory hallucinations. At times she grabs at imaginary things on her bed covers. Elsie tends to be rather resistive to nursing care and her fluid intake is poor. She is incontinent and constipated.

Using the problem-evaluation list develop a nursing care plan for this lady.

PROBLEM	NURSING CARE
Confused behaviour	
Anxiety/agitation	
Restlessness	
Resistiveness	
Diet	
General physical care	

18. Perhaps because of biorhythmic changes, or because of the reduction in environmental 'landmarks', or because of the use of sedation, patients are often more confused at night. It is 2 a.m. and Mr Bill F., aged 70, is awake and noisily calling out for 'Jean' [his wife]. When you get to his bedside he is in the process of getting up and asks you to get his clothes out as he is going to be late for work.

How would you handle this situation? Try to be specific.

19. Select a patient on your ward suffering from an acute confusional state.

i. What is the cause?

ii. List the diagnostic investigations carried out, giving the reasons for these tests.

iii. Describe the patient using the following headings:

Level of consciousness	Concentration
Activity level	Mood
Orientation/comprehension	Hallucinations/illusions/delusions

iv. Describe the nursing care of this patient showing how the problems indicated above were reduced/resolved.

We have tried to stress throughout this unit the importance of optimism and expectancy in caring for confused people. Improvement in mental clarity and social behaviour can be achieved with many patients given enthusiastic and appropriate medical and nursing care. One of the key aspects of the nurse's role with such patients is observation; not only to ensure safety but also with the aim of objectively assessing the patient's disabilities so that appropriate care and rehabilitation may be given.

20. Select a patient on your ward suffering from a confusional state, and using the rating scale below make an assessment of his current disabilities. Repeat your assessment towards the end of your placement or the patient's stay on the ward.

Discuss your involvement and responsibilities as a member of the treatment team in the care and rehabilitation of this patient. Indicate how you have been able to bring about any improvement highlighted by the rating scale.

Instructions: For each section please put a circle round the number that corresponds to the description that most suits the patient as he or she is now.

1. MOBILITY	5	Fully ambulant including stairs.
	4	Usually independent but not stairs.
	3	Walks with supervision.
	2	Walks with artificial aids or under careful supervision.
	1	Bedfast or chairfast most of the day.
2. ORIENTATION	5	Completely orientated.
	4	Orientated in ward and identifies persons correctly.
	3	Mis-identifies persons and surroundings but can find way about.
	2	Cannot find way to bed or toilet without assistance.
	1	Disorientated and gets lost.

3 COMMUNICATION	5	Always clear and retains information.
	4	Can indicate needs and understands directions; copes with information.
	3	Understands simple information but does not indicate needs.
	2	Cannot understand simple information; retains some expressive ability.
	1	No effective communication.
4. CO-OPERATION	5	Actively co-operative; offers to help.
	4	Passively co-operative; helps when asked.
	3	Willing but requires frequent encouragement.
	2	Rejects assistance and shows some independence.
	1	Completely resistive or withdrawn.
5. RESTLESSNESS	5	None.
	4	Intermittent.
	3	Persistent by day.
	2	Persistent by day with frequent nocturnal restlessness.
	1	Constant.
6. DRESSING	5	Dresses correctly unaided.
	4	Dressing imperfect but adequate.
	3	Dressing adequate with minimum supervision.
	2	Dressing inadequate unless continually supervised.
	1	Unable to dress or retain clothing because of mental impairment.
7. FEEDING	5	Feeds correctly and unaided at appropriate times.
	4	Feeds adequately with minimum supervision.

	3	Does not feed adequately unless continually supervised.
	2	Defective feeding due to physical handicap; poor appetite.
	1	Unable to feed because of mental impairment.
8. CONTINENCE	5	Fully continent.
	4	Nocturnal incontinence unless toileted; occasional accidents (urine or faeces).
	3	Continent by day if reguarly toileted.
	2	Urinary incontinence in spite of regular toileting.
	1	Regularly/frequently doubly incontinent.
9. HYGIENE	5	Washes without prompting.
	4	Needs reminding.
	3	Minimal supervision.
	2	Needs showing to the bathroom.
	1	Unable to wash without assistance.
10. SOCIABILITY	5	Very sociable, mixes well.
	4	Mixes well with own small circle of friends.
	3	Is a little wary of mixing.
	2	Withdrawn; very reluctant to converse.
	1	Unable to mix for physical or psychological reasons.
11. MOOD	5	Normal stable mood.
	4	Mild depression, anxiety, elation, aggression, lability.
	3	Moderate depression, anxiety, elation, aggression, lability.
	2	Severe depression, anxiety, elation, aggression, lability.

21. Mr Fred D. is 74 and suffers from senile dementia. He lives happily with his son and daughter-in-law who are both very fond of Fred. He is mildly confused and at times incontinent but can manage to dress and attend to his hygiene with a little assistance. Recently, however, he has been wandering at night, also occasionally during the day when his daughter-in-law has been at the shops. This has placed an additional burden on the family and has raised doubts about their ability to continue with the present arrangements.

i. What facilities exist to help support this patient in the community?
ii. Why is it desirable to continue to support this patient in the community?
iii. Outline the function of the psychogeriatric day hospital, emphasising the nurse's role.

A useful facility for elderly patients that has been established in some places is a crisis intervention service. This consists of a multidisciplinary team of personnel who are on call at all times throughout the week and will intervene at the request of a patient's GP to provide urgent medical assistance and supportive care in a psychiatric crisis. The object is to keep the patient out of hospital if at all possible and to treat the problem *in situ*. A person may be quietly confused or depressed for some time before his behaviour gets out of control and he becomes seriously disturbed, attracting the attention of others. Often this tenuous coping ability is undermined by a personal illness, the illness of a supporting relative, or increasing tension and the breakdown of goodwill within a family. Often these problems can be identified and resolved without the need for hospitalisation.

22. As a member of a crisis team called to assist with the following cases, outline the help the team might be able to provide.

The team, consisting of a doctor, nurse and social worker, are asked to visit Mr George P., aged 78, who lives in a small bungalow with his wife who is disabled and confined to a chair. The visit took place at 2.30 p.m. on Wednesday. Mrs P. reported that her husband had been rather muddled and forgetful for months, but recently everything seemed too much trouble for him and he had just lost interest and become very withdrawn. Mr P. appeared quite depressed and agitated and had obviously not washed or changed his clothes for days. There was no evidence of serious confusion. The house was in a neglected state and there was no food in the kitchen and no clean clothes for either of them to wear. Mrs P. had spent the previous night in the chair because her husband had been unable to help her to bed.

The team is called at 4.30 p.m. on Friday to visit Mrs Alice S. aged 82, who lives in a small terraced house by herself. She is looked after by her daughter who lives nearby. Recently her daughter had to go into hospital for an operation and since then the neighbours have been popping in. Although she has known them for years she has been behaving very oddly towards them over the past few days, accusing them of taking her pension and interfering with her belongings. Yesterday she drove them out of the house with a broom, saying she didn't know who they were or what they wanted. They are worried for her safety as she cannot cook for herself or attend to her hygiene unaided. On arrival at the house the team find Alice in a subdued but clearly confused state, mistaking one of the team for her brother. The house is cold; she obviously hasn't eaten recently and she has also been incontinent.

There has been much written about family life of old people and certainly the quality of life – the health, security and happiness of old people is closely bound up with the support and care they receive and the contribution they are able to make to family life. The view is common amongst nurses that families could and should do more for their ageing and infirm parents; that they have somehow jettisoned their moral obligations and have become less caring. There is no evidence that this is so. It should be remembered that a large elderly population is a comparatively new development and that changes in the size and mobility of families have made it difficult to provide supportive care. A study by Issacs (1971) into the reasons for admission of old people to a geriatric ward revealed that one-third were admitted for therapeutic optimism, one-third for lack of basic care (safety, food, cleanliness, warmth), and one-third because of the intolerable strain on their families. The majority of people in the group lacking in basic care were people with no close relatives.

23. The Briggs' live in a modern well-furnished three bedroomed semi on the outskirts of town. They have a daughter aged 14 and a son aged 19 who is away at college. Mr Briggs' mother has lived with them for the past two years and occupies the dining-room which has been converted into a bedroom for her use. Mrs Briggs (Senior) suffers from a mild degree of dementia, is muddled and forgetful and needs assistance with dressing, bathing and going to the toilet. She is a rather demanding and overdependent lady who plays on her son's rather doting attitude. Mrs Briggs (Junior) feels she has had enough. She thinks her mother-in-law has caused tension between her and her husband and feels that she deserves a life of her own now the children are growing up. Mr Briggs has always been very close to his mother and tends to fuss over her. He tends to be a little unsympathetic and unsupportive towards his wife. Sally Briggs is fond of her Gran, but notices how moody her mother has become just lately and she resents having to stay in and sit with Gran; she also feels frustrated that she cannot bring her friends back.

Explore further the attitudes, feelings and frustrations of the individual members of this family.

24. The continued support of relatives is vital to the morale and individuality of elderly patients hospitalised.

Discuss the needs and problems of the relatives of such patients and suggest ways in which support may be given and goodwill and involvement encouraged.

NURSING THE ELDERLY
Self Evaluation Test

1. Select from the list below the three most common psychiatric disorders found in the elderly:

a. schizophrenia;
b. arteriosclerotic dementia;
c.. depression;
d. phobic anxiety;
e. Huntington's chorea;
f. acute confusional state.

2. Select from he list below two clinical features that are commonly found in dementia:

a. thought blocking;
b. retardation;
c. amnesia;
d. emotional incongruity;
e. confabulation.

3. In the care of elderly patients the ward environment should be:

a. restful and relaxing;
b. comfortable and warm;
c. socially and mentally stimulating;
d. Safe
(i) d.
(ii) c, d
(iii) a, b, d
(iv) all of the above.

4. Disinhibition is a common feature of dementia which leads to . . .
Select the best response from the list below:

a. confused behaviour;
b. coarsening of social behaviour;
c. excitable overactive behaviour;
d. social withdrawal.

5. Loss of interest, retardation, poor concentration, personal neglect, constipation are clinical features of . . .
Select the best response from the list below.

a. institutionalisation;
b. dementia;
c. schizophrenia;
d. depression.

6. Common causes of urinary incontinence in the elderly are . . .
Select the two most appropriate responses from the list below:

a. nephritis;
b. damage to spinal cord;
c. Normal ageing;
d. loss of cortical inhibition;
e. disorientation.

7. An elderly confused patient with a respiratory infection begins to get dressed and says he is going to work. In *most* cases would you:

a. take his clothes away and put up cot-sides;
b. tell him firmly to stay in bed;
c. ask the doctor to prescribe some sedation;
d. try to increase his orientation.

8. Disorientation is a mental disability in which a person:

a. experiences hallucinations;
b. is unable to recall events;
c. loses ability to accurately appreciate time, place, person;
d. experiences difficulty in answering simple questions.

9. Social isolation in old age may be caused by . . .
Select the best response from the list below:

a. loss of mobility;
b. personality defects;
c. deafness;
d. bereavement;
e. retirement.
(i) a, c
(ii) d,
(iii) a, b, c, d
(iv) all of the above.

10. Select from the list below three clinical features that are commonly found in acute confusional states:

a. restlessness;
b. flight of ideas;
c. hallucinations;
d. apprehension;
e. emotional incongruity;
f. perseveration.

Assertion and reason

Each of the questions in this section consists of an assertion followed by a reason. Assign to each question one of the five categories (a – e) given in the key below:

KEY

a. The assertion and reason are both true.
The reason is a correct explanation of the assertion.
b. The assertion and reason are both true.
The reason is *not* a correct explanation of the assertion.
c. The assertion is true but the reason is false.
d. The assertion is false but the reason is true.
e. The assertion and reason are both false.

ASSERTION
1. Depression often accompanies arteriosclerotic dementia.

REASON
The centres of the brain concerned with emotion are damaged.

ASSERTION
2. Admitting to hospital elderly patients with dementia may increase their confusion.

REASON
The risk of developing an infection is increased.

ASSERTION
3. These days elderly people in our society enjoy a much improved standard of mental health.

REASON
They are well integrated with the community and have a valued social role.

ASSERTION
4. Patients with dementia may behave in an aggressive paranoid way.

REASON
Impaired memory causes people to misinterpret situations.

ASSERTION
5. People with a history of Huntington's chorea should not have children.

REASON
The disease is carried by a dominant gene.

ASSERTION
6. The geriatric nurse should never do for the patients what the patient can do for themselves.

REASON
Promotes dependent and regressive behaviour and causes a lowering in morale.

ASSERTION
7. Extreme restlessness often accompanies confused behaviour.

REASON
General inactivity and anxiety are commonly experienced by hospitalised patients.

ASSERTION
8. Following ECT patients often have no recollection of having had treatment.

REASON
Long-term memory is very vulnerable to distruption and loss.

ASSERTION
9. Families nowadays have a less caring attitude towards their ageing relatives.

REASON
Changes in the size and mobility of families have made it more difficult to provide supportive care.

ASSERTION
10. Confusion is often worse at night.

REASON
Surroundings are less familiar in the subdued light.

ASSERTION
11. The acutely confused patient should be nursed in quiet, well-lit surroundings.

REASON
Sensory deprivation increases confused behaviour.

True/False items

1. Suicide is common amongst men in the 65+ age-group. (True; False)
2. Social isolation is an important contributory factor in depression and suicide. (True; False)
3. Social devaluation means being forced to accept a lower standard of living. (True; False)
4. Dysphasia is the inability to articulate and express words clearly. (True; False)
5. The long-term memory is affected in the early stages of dementia. (True; False)

6. Pathological changes in mood are a prominent feature of cerebral syphilis. (True; False)
7. Mental clarity may be improved by a simple consistent day-to-day routine. (True; False)
8. Delirium is confusion of a progressive and permanent nature. (True; False)
9. More women than men suffer from senile dementia. (True; False)
10. Epileptiform seizures often occur in chronic confusional states. (True; False)
11. People remember only what they want to remember. (True; False)

REFERENCES AND FURTHER READING

Agate, J. (1972), *Geriatrics for Nurses and Social Workers*, Heinemann.
Burneside, I. (1976), *Nursing the Aged*, McGraw-Hill.
Bromley, D. (1974), *The Psychology of Human Ageing*, Pelican.
Carver, V. (ed.) (1978), *An Ageing Population*, Hodder & Stoughton.
Hilgard, R., Atkinson, R. C., and Atkinson, R. L. (1975), *Introduction to Psychology*, 6th edition, Harcourt Brace Jovanovich.
Issacs, B. (1971), *Survival of the unfittest: Study of Geriatric Patients in Glasgow*.
McGhie, A. (1979), *Psychology as Applied to Nursing*, Churchill Livingstone.
Pitt, B. (1978), *Psycho-Geriatrics*, Churchill Livingstone.
Whitehead, D. (1978), *In the Service of Old Age*, H.M. &M. Publications.
——(1979), *Psychiatric Disorder in Old Age*, H.M. & M. Publications.

Unit 7

Nursing Patients Dependent on Drugs and Alcohol

INTRODUCTION

The abuse of alcohol and other drugs is a major health problem in this country. As a society we moralise about the effects of excessive drinking, penalise the drinker's transgressions of the law, and express concern and dismay at the increase of drug abuse amongst our children. Yet we are a nation of pill-takers and drinkers and, by our example, make acceptable the principle of the habitual use of drugs and alcohol.

Although much of the therapeutic work with addicts is carried out in special units, the nurse will come across the problem of drug abuse in many different situations. The barbiturate addict admitted to casualty following an overdose, the middle-aged lady in the community dosing herself with transquillisers, the man with alcohol polyneuritis on the medical ward, and the young man admitted to the psychiatric unit with a drug-induced psychosis, are a few examples.

The aims of this unit are to help the nurse to develop a more informed, sensitive, helpful approach to drug dependent patients, and to become a more effective member of the treatment team.

THE CARE OF PATIENTS DEPENDENT ON ALCOHOL

> If all be true that I do think,
> There are five good reasons we should drink;
> Good wine – a friend – or being dry –
> Or lest we should be by and by
> Or any other reason why.
>
> Henry Aldrich

As the rhyme light-heartedly points out, any reason is good enough to drink. Every day millions of people drink alcohol, a drug, and enjoy doing so. It has an accepted place in our culture, yet our relationship with alcohol is an uneasy one, for much ill health, unhappiness and crime results from its consumption. This uneasiness is reflected in society's rather ambivalent attitude to drinking. The man who can 'hold his drink' acquires a certain status in his social group – it is regarded as an attribute of masculinity, and yet the drunk is often seen as a figure of fun, his actions providing much material for comedians and cartoonists. So a society that tolerates and even encourages the use of a drug that reduces self-control, may well condemn and punish such loss of control when it causes embarrassment and lawbreaking.

1. Many people regard alchoholism as a sign of self-indulgence and moral weakness. How would you counter this attitude?

2. Compare the effects of the following drugs:
alcohol barbiturates heroin.

Many attempts have been made to define alcohol-dependence. Of these two are generally accepted as being the most satisfactory.

3. Find the WHO definition of alcohol-dependence (1952) and compare this with the definition produced by Keller (1960).

The phenomenon of dependence is described as being either physical or psychological in nature, or both.

4. Differentiate between these two types of dependence.
i. Psychological
ii. Physical.

5. Kessel and Walton (1967) identify three stages in the development of alcoholism. Briefly describe these stages.
i. Excessive drinking
ii. The dependence stage
iii. Chronic alcoholism.

Professor Jellinek (1960) considers alcoholism to be a generic term including five types of alcoholism.

6. Complete the classification of alcoholism according to Professor Jellinek:
Alpha
Beta
Gamma
Delta
Epsilon

It is difficult to arrive at an accurate figure for the number of persons dependent on alcohol in the population. The difference between excessive drinking and alcohol-dependence is often arbitrary, the reluctance on the part of persons to admit to the disease being an added difficulty.

An estimate by the Office of Health Economics in 1970 using the WHO definition and based on several reliable sources, was of between 200,000 and 400,000 persons dependent on alcohol in England and Wales. This is supported by the National Council of Alchoholism who, in 1977, reported an estimated eleven adults in every 1000 as having a drink problem.

Several theories have been suggested attempting to identify causative factors in alcoholism.

7. Below is a list of these factors. Describe each briefly:

physiological	psychoanalytical
psychological vulnerability	occupational
learning (behaviourists') theory	social and cultural

From figures compiled by the Registrar General, it would appear that excessive drinking is a greater health problem amongst the higher social groups.

8. Comment on the significance of this.

In recent years changes have occurred regarding the incidence of alcohol-dependence in relation to age and sex. Traditionally alcoholism has been seen as a problem amongst men in the middle age group. There is now a fast-growing problem of alcoholism, often in association with other types of drug abuse, amongst the young of both sexes in this country.

9. What reasons can you find for the change described above?

In addition alcoholism amongst older women is also on the increase, particularly in the higher social classes.

At the onset of the disease the alcohol temporarily relieves the sufferer's problems and reduces tension. Inevitably, however, the alcohol impairs the drinker's normal functioning, which in turn causes a further increase in tension, necessitating the need for more alcohol. A truly vicious circle!

Heavy drinkers tend to gravitate to spirits rather than beer. The type of drink used is immaterial, since both are merely vehicles to carry the alcohol. However, as the alcohol content is much higher in spirits than in beer, obviously a much smaller quantity is required to achieve the desired effect.

As a person's need for alcohol exceeds the purchasing power of his income, he/she will resort to other methods to raise the necessary money, often these people deprive themselves and their families of other essentials.

10. Describe the methods such a person may have to resort to, in order to continue drinking.

11. Consider the stress and conflicts that may exist within the family of a heavy drinker.

In the early stages, most excessive drinkers drink in the same pattern as moderate social drinkers, but steadily drink more. That is, their drinking is usually confined at first to public houses and at parties, but their intake is greater than that of their social group. This period of increasing drinking varies greatly in length; Professor Jellinek suggested anything from three to twenty years.

As the disease progresses, the sufferer's drinking becomes furtive and more private, they prefer their own company because of their companions' inability or lack of desire to drink at the increased rate. As their demand increases they develop strategies to ensure a constant supply of alcohol.

12. What strategies might the excessive drinker resort to in order to ensure a constantly available supply?

The drinking continues and worsens, and the need for alcohol is increased by a developing tolerance to its effects, a greater consumption being required to achieve the same relief. When the excessive drinker reaches the point where alcohol is a continual necessity, he/she is now dependent on the drug.

For mental health workers, the greatest single problem in helping persons dependent on alcohol is their reluctance to recognise and admit their need for help. This is important, as the basis of successful treatment is the acceptance by the patient of the part alcohol has played in causing his problems, and genuine motivation to overcome these problems by controlling the drinking.

Defence mechanisms are frequently used by alcoholics to explain their drinking and its effects, and to lessen their sense of guilt and anxiety.

13. Give examples of how the following mechanisms might be used:
rationalisation projection denial.

Alcohol, as well as being a drug, is also a poison, and its continued usage to excess will eventually have a detrimental effect on the body. In addition to its toxic effects on the liver causing cirrhosis, it produces pathological changes in the brain which may lead to intellectual deterioration.

14. During this stage of dependence blackouts become a feature of the disease.

- **i.** Describe the form these blackouts usually take.
- **ii.** What methods does the sufferer use in an attempt to disguise these episodes?

As the disease progresses further alcoholics lose the ability to control their drinking at all. Their only interest in life is alcohol and they often become abusive and aggressive when attempts are made to modify their behaviour. Their work deteriorates and they frequently lose their jobs. Their already strained family relationships are stretched to breaking point and they may well become pathologically jealous of their spouse. They become isolated, remorseful and despairing. Understandably suicide attempts are not uncommon. In spite of all this, they are often the last ones to recognise the real cause of their condition. This is the state in which they are so often admitted to hospital.

15. Select a patient admitted to your unit following a lengthy bout of intoxication.

i. Identify the physical effects of his drinking.
ii. Describe the treatment régime that was used to remedy these effects.

One problem which may be encountered following admission is that of withdrawal symptoms. These may occur within several hours or even several days of the cessation of drinking. Occasionally they may take the form of delirium tremens in which the patient is very restless, trembles uncontrollably, sweats and may have seizures. Consciousness is usually clouded and the patient disorientated and confused, often experiencing visual hallucinations and illusions of a terrifying nature. Persecutory delusions may also be present. The use of therapeutic measures such as Vitamin B complex and chlormethiazole (Heminevrin) have made such episodes rare events today. More commonly mild withdrawal states are seen in which the patient may suffer from the shakes, feel mildly confused and generally unwell.

You may find it helpful at this point to refer to the unit on nursing the confused patient, which deals with the nursing care of patients in acute confusional states.

16. A problem that might be encountered when caring for the alcoholic patient, is that of continued drinking after admission.

A patient returns to the unit in a noisy and truculent state. He has obviously been drinking.

i. What would be your immediate reaction and how would you manage the situation?
ii. How might this episode affect your relationship with the patient?
iii. What action may the treatment team/ward community take following such an incident?

Simply condemning a patient's drinking habits will only serve to reinforce his guilt feelings and may even increase them. A complete cessation of drinking is considered essential by some, but forced abstinence based on the patient's guilt feelings or fear of the consequences is unlikely to be successful. For treatment to result in a permanent adjustment to a life in which the intake of alcohol is controlled, or abstained from completely, the patient has to be faced with the reality of their situation and behaviour.

17. Select a patient on your unit who has been recently admitted with a drink problem. What clues are there in his conversation and behaviour to suggest that he is not facing reality?

Confronting the patient with reality in order that he might gain an insight into his condition is usually an emotionally painful process. The patient is faced with problems his drinking has caused for himself and for others, and the disturbance that has resulted in his life. Such sessions may be carried out in a one-to-one situation, but are usually most effective in the group situation.

18. What role may the following groups play in confrontation sessions:

i. A small 'closed' ward group
ii. Alcoholics Anonymous (AA)
iii. A small 'confrontation' group including the patient's employer, a close friend and his wife?

Patients frequently become remorseful and depressed following reality-confrontation sessions. It is necessary for self-confidence and self-esteem to be restored and guilt feelings ventilated. This can be done either in a group situation or in a one-to-one relationship with the nurse.

19. Describe how in your nursing approach you could help raise the patient's self-esteem and restore optimism about the future. Be specific.

Group therapy is the usual treatment of choice. In addition to being a vehicle for reality confrontation, ventilation of feelings and a source of support and encouragement the group can help the alcoholic face and resolve underlying personality problems that may have been masked by his drinking for many years.

20. Briefly describe the following treatment regimes:

i. Aversion therapy
ii. Antabuse (Disulfiram) therapy.

Alcoholism has been described as a family disease because of the effect it has on the stability and security of the family unit. An intact family and a helpful and understanding spouse is considered one of the best prognostic factors.

Mrs Jane Y., married with two children, has suffered the stresses and strains of her husband's excessive drinking for eight years. Although he is now in hospital for treatment she has no confidence in his assurances that he will 'never touch another drop'. Mrs Y., says she can no longer put up with his dishonesty and total lack of concern for the family's welfare. She has isolated him from her affections and from all family responsibilities.

21. How might you help Jane towards a more positive attitude to her husband's problem?

22. What part might the following agencies play in supporting this family whilst he is in hospital:

i. The social worker
ii. Al Anon

The need for alcohol has been a major part of an alcoholic's life prior to treatment, and the removal of alcohol will leave a 'vacuum' that is difficult to fill. The patient's life-style may well have to alter to avoid obvious temptation to drink. Previously strained or broken relationships may have to be repaired and readjusted and an attempt made to engender trust. New hobbies and interests will need to be fostered, or old ones rekindled, and overall an effort must be made to help the patient regain his lost social prestige. This process of rehabilitation begins in hospital but it is most important that it should continue following discharge.

23. What support should the following offer during this difficult period:

i. The patient's spouse and immediate family
ii. The psychiatric day hospital
iii. The hospital-based community nurse?

The more traditional approach of complete abstinence has been questioned in recent years. In several units in this country patients are helped to learn to control their drinking, rather than to abstain completely. Total abstinence is considered an unrealistic goal for many patients and therefore would be an obstacle to effective therapy. To be allowed to continue drinking, but to have to learn to control the amount and frequency, is considered by many patients more attainable and more dignified.

It is not a method that would be suitable for all patients. An accurate assessment is made by the treatment team and two criteria must be fulfilled. It must be shown that the patients physical condition allows them to continue drinking in a controlled manner; and secondly, the patient must choose controlled drinking as his treatment goal.

The treatment principles are behavioural, aimed at changing learned drinking patterns. Specialized behavioural procedures are used and nurses involved in this approach require a sound knowledge of behaviour modification techniques.

Following education about their problem and the treatment, patients are introduced to techniques enabling them to control their rate of drinking. Additionally, they are helped to develop social and relaxation skills as alternatives to drinking during periods of increased difficulty.

Pre-disposing social and occupational factors are altered where possible, and family support is encouraged as patients attempt to transfer their new skills from the treatment unit to the home environment. Often patients are encouraged to complete a 'behavioural diary' relating to their drinking patterns following discharge, and this aids the community nurse to support and monitor their continued progress.

24. Consider what is meant by the statement 'An alcoholic is always only one drink away from a relapse'.
Discuss with your group whether the implications in the above statement can be reconciled with the concept of controlled drinking.

The final stage in this disorder, if it is not halted, is that of chronic alcoholism. This is marked by the development of additional physical and psychiatric disorders. Medical advice is frequently sought for such physical disorders as peripheral neuritis, cardiomyopathy and heptatic cirrhosis.

Malnutrition, and in particular a deficiency of vitamin B_1 (thiamine) may lead to a brain disturbance known as Wernicke's encephalopathy. This is characterised by confusion, memory impairment and ataxia.

It is not unusual in chronic alcoholism for an alcoholic psychosis to occur. This is known as Korsakoff's (Korsakov or dysmnesic) syndrome. The most marked feature of this disorder is memory loss for recent events and confabulation. In addition, the patient is frequently disorientated, labile and suggestible. The onset is usually insidious, but may follow an attack of delirium tremens or Wernicke's encephalopathy.

Personality changes are common in all forms of chronic alcoholism. Judgement becomes poor, emotional changes such as lability, irritability or euphoria may occur and general control of the environment is impaired.

During the final stages of the disease tolerance to alcohol frequently diminishes. The alcoholics' loss of social stability and status often ends in their drinking methylated spirit or other impure alcohol substitutes and living rough as vagrants and outcasts; a state that further hastens their already marked physical and mental decline.

A proportion of alcoholics eventually suffer from dementia. The mood-changes of chronic alcoholism become worse, a flattened effect being characteristic, coupled with apathy. As with other types of dementia, the patients are confused, disorientated, particularly for place and time, their social behaviour deteriorates, and they frequently become totally dependent on the Institution.

You may find it useful at this point to refer to the Unit 'The care of the Confused Patient', that deals with the care of the patient with dementia.

25. Either select a patient on your unit suffering from alcoholism or use the following case-summary to complete a care-treatment programme emphasising the nursing involvement using the evaluative list of needs.

Dave E., aged 38, married, with one child, is admitted to your unit with a history of alcohol-dependence. Dave lost his job as an engineer four months ago because of his deteriorating work performance, and now his marriage seems to be in danger of breaking up because of his excessive drinking. He has come into hospital reluctantly, under pressure from his wife and GP following a lengthy bout of intoxication and self-neglect. Dave claims he can control his drinking, and says the reason he has been drinking a lot lately is that he has been going through a bad patch. Dave has always had a deep sense of personal inadequacy and has never quite measured up to his expectations of himself. Alcohol has in the past helped him experience a sense of personal worth and confidence.

PROBLEM	NURSING CARE
Possible medical complications.	
Management during withdrawal phase.	
Unable to face the reality of his problem.	
Lacks desire and confidence to stop drinking.	
Coping with guilt feelings, despondency and frustration.	
To develop self-acceptance and personality growth.	
Social rehabilitation.	

CARE OF PATIENTS DEPENDENT ON DRUGS

At some time in their lives virtually everyone has taken drugs. The way in which the drug is taken, and the general attitudes towards the drug, can be divided into three groups.

The first group contains those drugs which society has come to think of as desirable and harmless; so much so in fact that they are not usually called drugs. If you smoke then you have taken nicotine, 'a mood-changer'. When you drink tea, coffee, cocoa, or even Coca-cola you are taking caffeine, a stimulant. Alcohol, as was shown earlier in the unit, is also a most potent mood-changer and appears to act both as a 'stimulant' and soporific (although of course alcohol is a CNS depressant).

In the second group are those drugs that are also patent 'mood-changers', but are not accepted by society as being desirable or harmless. For this reason the sale or possession of such drugs is illegal. Heroin and the other opiates; cocaine, cannabis (either as marijuana or hashish) and LSD fall into this group. The latter drug is not regarded as a 'mood-changer' as such, but more as a 'mind-bender'.

Drugs that are prescribed by doctors for treatment, or those purchased from chemists for the purpose of self-treatment, constitute the third group. It would be almost impossible to estimate the number of drugs bought over the chemists' counter during any one year.

An individual may become dependent on any of the drugs in these three categories.

26. Discuss the reasons for the different social attitudes to drugs in these three categories.

Drug abuse is considered to have taken place when, with the exception of drugs prescribed by a doctor for the treatment of physical or mental ill health, they are taken solely for the mood-changing or mind-bending effects. The abuser becomes increasingly dependent on the drug and is unable voluntarily to discontinue taking it.

Such abuse is not limited to one drug only. Different drugs are frequently mixed and taken in the form of a 'cocktail' and the growing trend for alcoholism to occur in association with the abuse of other drugs, particularly amongst the young, is cause for concern.

27. Commonly abused drugs are categorised by their effect. Describe the general effect of the following, giving examples of drugs in each group:

sedatives
stimulants
narcotics
tranquillisers
hallucinogens

On occasions less known substances are abused and may reflect passing fads in adolescent subcultures. Below is given a list of such substances:

modelling glue
lacquer
lighter fuel
Morning Glory seeds
cough linctus

The causes of drug abuse and dependence bear many similarities to that of alcoholism.

28. Below is given a list of factors that may be influential in causing drug abuse and dependence. Comment on each.

occupation
experimentation
peer group pressure
psychological vulnerability
availability

29. What evidence is there to suggest that the abuse of the so-called 'soft-drugs', for example, cannabis, may cause graduation onto 'hard drugs' such as heroin.

One causative factor not present in alcoholism is abuse following the legitimate prescription of a drug. Abuse of narcotics, following prescription for severe pain or post-operative use, can occur. However, the awareness among the medical profession of this danger, and the availability of less addictive substances, has led to a decrease in the number of people becoming dependent in this way. Another example of how the medical profession may influence and control abuse is the voluntary ban imposed in the UK on the prescription of amphetamines, a drug which was widely abused in the early 1960s, often as the result of indiscriminate over-prescribing.

There is evidence that a similar awareness to the dangers of barbiturate-prescribing is leading to a voluntary ban with regard to this drug, in certain parts of the country. However, it is estimated that one billion anti-depressants and minor tranquillisers were taken between 1964 and 1967. Recent evidence seems to indicate that this rate of administration has not decreased, and it is thus understandable that a proportion of these legitimate users should become dependent on such drugs. In addition, it was reported in 1978 that a growing problem was that of people being introduced to the drug habit by relatives or friends, who 'shared' their legitimately prescribed medication with them.

In early response to the growing concern in this country during the early 1960s about the escalating 'drug problem' a committee was set up under the chairmanship of Lord Brain. In its report, published in 1965, were recommendations aimed at establishing control of drugs and these were embodied in the Dangerous Drug Act of 1967. This act was superseded by the Misuse of Drugs Act 1971 which came into force in 1973.

30. Comment on each of the following, indicating what effect they have had on the pattern and scale of the drug problem in this country.
- **i.** Notification of addicts
- **ii.** Treatment centres
- **iii.** Reclassification of commonly abused drugs.

Since the drugs of abuse are strictly controlled, the would-be abuser usually has to resort to an illegal supply of the drug. The supplier is often called a 'pusher' and his services are naturally expensive. Pushers are frequently dependent on drugs themselves and they operate in the twilight zone between the normal and criminal worlds. They are usually no more than a link between the real supplier and the addict, their aim being to increase their trade in order to maintain their own supply. Many young addicts, however, supply each other with drugs, and when one has a plentiful supply, perhaps from a chemist break-in, he will supply his friends on the understanding that the friends will reciprocate when they in turn obtain drugs, or 'score', as it is called.

31. What may be the social consequences for the addict of having to obtain drugs illegally through a street pusher?

Drug abuse is often associated with a sub-culture of its own. In some senses it is a secretive culture, yet conversely members of it feel the need to advertise their membership by adopting a distinctive form of dress, taste in music and the arts and a very definite set of anti-establishment attitudes. As with many other sub-cultures the use of slang gives an element of exclusiveness, yet further advertises its existence.

32. Describe what is meant by the following terms.

connexion	blocked
fix	a trip (good or bad)

joint
mainline, shoot
busted
cold turkey
head *or* freak
pop, popping

33. In the same way commonly abused drugs are given nicknames. Give the correct name or type of drug for the following:

snow, coke, Charlie
H, horse, smack
M, Emma
hot and cold speedballs
pot, grass, weed, tea, shit
hash
bennies
speed, hearts, Frenchies
goof balls, sleepers
purple haze, acid

There are two important aspects in the treatment and nursing care of the drug-dependent patient.

First, the immediate or short-term objectives. This involves the emergency treatment of accidental or deliberate overdose; and the relief of physical dependence by medically supervised withdrawal of the drug.

Secondly, the long-term objectives. This includes psychological and social rehabilitation directed towards helping the addict make the necessary adjustments in his/her life.

In recent years amphetamine has been a very popular drug of abuse. Overall the effect is to act as a stimulant, producing feelings of euphoria and great energy and alertness in the user. When taken intravenously users describe the initial feeling (the 'rush' or 'flash') as resembling a complete body orgasm. It is a matter of debate whether physical dependence and consequently withdrawal symptoms occur with amphetamine abuse. Certainly users suffer from a 'hangover' depression when the effects wear off. Psychological dependence is severe and prolonged abuse may result in a toxic psychosis occurring. The clinical picture often resembles that of paranoid schizophrenia, especially in persons with an immature unstable personality. They may be very restless and confused but the dominant feature is of paranoid delusions, ideas of reference, and hallucinations.

A comparison of the effects of barbiturates with those of alcohol has been made earlier in the unit. Barbituric acid and other hypnotics are the most commonly abused drugs. Its effects on the user are extrememly destructive and equal to that of heroin in terms of personality changes; the withdrawal effects are probably more severe.

34. Describe the physical complications that may accompany the withdrawal of barbiturates following prolonged use of large doses.

In an effort to reduce the likelihood of these complications, barbiturates are withdrawn slowly, the dosage often being reduced by 100 mg/day.

With both amphetamine and barbiturate-dependence, anxiety and insomnia may be present at some stage in the illness.

35. How could these problems be best managed by the treatment team, remembering the patient's strong dependency needs?

Opium and its derivatives, morphine and heroin (diamorphine) constitute a group of highly potent drugs of abuse. Heroin is potentially more dangerous than morphine and the prognosis for such dependence is bad. The methods of administration of heroin are by injection, either intravenously or subcutaneously, or by being sniffed ('snorted'). The only fixed events in a heroin addict's day are to obtain and administer a dose of the drug. Life revolves around this point and motivation for anything else is lost, inevitably leading to self-neglect and eventual social degradation.

36. **i.** List the physical complications of long-term abuse of heroin.
ii. Consider how these will be managed by the treatment team.

The withdrawal of opiates, and heroin in particular, produces severe and very unpleasant side-effects. Again for this reason, the drug is withdrawn slowly over a period of days, and a substitute drug is usually given. Methadone (Physeptone), a synthetic analgesic with opiate-like effects, is generally used, and on occasions codeine may be substituted. In addition, these may be accompanied by the administration of Valium and Librium. In some units, prolonged narcosis has been used during the withdrawal stage.

37. List the features of a medically unsupervised withdrawal from heroin.

The hallucinogenic drugs, ranging from the more potent mescaline and lysergic acid diethylamide (LSD) to the less potent cannabis sativa are increasingly abused in this country. It has been estimated that as many as four million people have experimented with cannabis in one form or another.

38. A patient has a history of taking cannabis regularly. He/she asks you why it shouldn't be legalised, saying that its effects are no worse than alcohol.

There is said to be no danger of physical dependence with these drugs, but psychological dependence does occur. They enhance sensory perception, produce a state of unreality and depersonalisation, and stimulate hallucinations. It is the hallucinations, more than anything, that provides the attraction with LSD. The user may state that he can 'see' music or 'hear' colours, and that 'visions' give a new meaning to life. The hallucinations may be incredibly beautiful or intensely frightening and horrific. Unfortunately the effects of the drug cannot be predicted prior to ingestion. The effects of a 'bad trip' can last for months and even produce a severe psychotic state.

It should be noted that the withdrawal stage is an excellent opportunity for the nurse to begin to build a therapeutic relationship with the patient; a relationship that will be vital during the rehabilitative period.

The attitude of the treatment team towards the drug-dependent patient is a vital factor in the overall treatment programme. The relapse rate is high amongst discharged addicts and their period of hospitalisation is often marked by disruptive and manipulative behaviour and episodes of illicit drug consumption. For these reasons the prevailing attitude might well be one of pessimism and cynicism. This is unhelpful and often self-defeating, and may well produce an oversimplistic and rigid attitude to treatment and nursing care.

It is essential that the treatment teams have an optimistic, sympathetic yet firm approach to the patient. Consistency is vital and team meetings must decide management principles for each patient. Staff must be able to freely ventilate their feelings and resolve disagreements. Disruptive patients will soon sense strain amongst the treatment team and will quickly exploit the situation.

39. Discuss with the group your personal attitudes towards the drug-dependent patient.

40. Entering the bathroom you find Andy V., hiding a bottle of Tuinal capsules in the lavatory cistern. You felt you had previously established a good relationship with Andy and are surprised and disappointed by his behaviour. He asks you not to report him to the treatment team and insists he is only holding them for a friend who will collect them the next day. Andy says he feels he can trust you and that you are the only person that really understands his problem.

How would you deal with this situation? Be specific.

The relationship between the nurse and the addict may greatly influence the process of rehabilitation. Addicts frequently have high dependency needs and lean heavily on such a relationship for support and encouragement in the early stages of treatment. Through this relationship the addict may ventilate his feelings and frustrations and explore his attitudes and problems. He may identify strongly with the nurse, using him/her as a role model for more mature behaviour.

41. How might you use your relationship with a young heroin addict to help him try and resolve the following problems?

to cope more successfully with frustrations
to relate more successfully to authority
to confront the reality of his dependence
to maintain a positive desire and the confidence to stay off drugs
to improve his self-esteem and optimism?

Complete stabilisation of the person dependent on drugs may take as long as six to twelve months. When primary withdrawal has been successfully completed, psychological and social rehabilitation can begin in earnest. The major task is maintaining abstention during the period of social and psychological adjustment. Often drugs have represented a defence between individuals and their problems. Once stripped of this defence they feel threatened and vulnerable and their resolve to abstain weakens. Individual and group psychotherapy is used extensively to help resolve these underlying personality problems.

It is also important to realise that often the drug becomes 'all things' to the addict and represents the only source of pleasure and satisfaction. Whilst on drugs personal and sexual relationships become redundant and the addict feels little need to explore his intellectual or creative potential. Therefore, little personality growth takes place during the addictive phase.

During the course of dependence the addict may well have 'opted out' socially, and equally the community may well have rejected him. Patients with drug problems are frequently unemployed, homeless and without money or friends. They often drift away from their families and lead squalid existences in the decaying areas of the big cities. Drug abuse is frequently more than just a disorder; it is a way of life, and the great vacuum created by the absence of drugs from their lives presents a challenging obstacle in rehabilitation.

John F., aged 21, is an intelligent young man from a working class background in a provincial town. He has been an addict using a variety of drugs since he was 17. During this time he has had a number of unskilled jobs for short periods and has now lost contact with his family. John has known no other life but talking about, obtaining and using drugs for the last three years. His only 'friends' are other addicts.

42. Consider how you might help John develop new sources of interest and pleasure.

43. Consider how the treatment team might help John re-establish himself in the community.

One of the problems associated with treating drug-dependent patients in hospital is that the social environment of the treatment is 'unreal' in relation to the world outside and may foster dependency and the development of unrealistic attitudes. A further disadvantage is that in specialised units the prevailing attitude amongst a group of addicts may become negative and anti-therapeutic as drug experiences are shared and group identity established.

44. Consider the advantages and disadvantages of treating the drug-dependent patient (including alcoholics) in the community.

45. Select a patient on your unit who has been admitted suffering from barbituarate-dependence. Draw up a nursing care plan to meet the needs of this patient.

OR Using the following case history write your care plan:

Tony B., aged 38, has been on the unit for 36 hours following admission resulting from prolonged barbiturate intoxication. He has been taking approximately 1.2g of sodium amytal daily for several months. He is a clerical officer in a large manufacturing company and he first took the drug during a particularly difficult period at work. At that time his company was going through a bad time and there were rumours of redundancy circulating amongst the staff. Tony felt that his job was particularly vulnerable and became more and more anxious and distressed about his future. His wife had previously been prescribed sodium amytal to help her sleep, and Tony decided to take one to calm himself down. He began to increasingly depend on them and, even when his fears about his future were shown to be groundless, he was unable to stop taking them. In fact he had to resort to complaining to his GP of insomnia to supplement his wife's supply of the drug. It was only when his GP became suspicious of the frequency of visits to his surgery that, on questioning Tony's wife, the truth emerged. His GP advised admission to hospital.

On admission Tony was weepy and depressed and his personal appearance indicated neglect of personal hygiene. He had been unable to work for several weeks, and his wife stated at most times his mood was very unpredictable, changing daily from irritability to one of amusement and light-heartedness. On other occasions he was suspicious and aggressive, particularly with strangers, and she expressed great concern over his recent accusations that their two children were the result of previous extra-marital affairs by his wife. His physical condition is beginning to cause concern for the staff.

46. Simon D., aged 23, has been admitted to the unit having taken an unspecified amount of LSD. Two days ago, Simon was found wandering down the centre of a busy street in a 'trance-like' state wrapped only in a blanket. On admission he is restless and excited. He says he is in communication with God and that he can walk through walls.

Describe the approach you would use in the initial management of this patient. Be specific.

As the above case-summary indicates, one of the dangers associated with taking LSD is that a protracted psychotic state may be induced. This is particularly so if the individual is psychologically vulnerable, for example being in a depressed state before taking the drug, or having a history of psychotic illness, or if the inexperienced person takes the drug unsupervised by more experienced friends.
What other dangers are associated with taking hallucinogenic drugs?

47. Select a patient on your unit who has been admitted following multiple abuse of drugs. Using the criteria given, construct a nursing care plan.

OR Construct your plan using the following case-history:

Sandra S., aged 20, has been admitted to your unit as a condition of her probation following a shop-lifting offence. She has been 'living rough' for several weeks and is obviously suffering from malnutrition and gross personal neglect. Injection scars and abscesses are present on both arms. Sandra is an intelligent girl and comes from a 'middle class' family background. She has an elder married brother, and a younger sister at home. She left home two years ago following protracted arguments with her father about her friends, and what were, in his opinion, her 'weird' interests and activities. Apart from an occasional visit to her mother shortly after leaving, she has not been home since. She started taking barbiturates and amphetamines about 14 months ago when offered some by a friend. At that time she had just split up with her current boy-friend and was feeling particularly lonely and unhappy. About a year ago she gave up her job as a window-dresser and has not worked since. She began taking heroin a year ago and became notified as an addict six months later. Sandra has been receiving a daily dose of 20 mg of physeptone by prescription and she supplements this with illicit barbiturates and heroin when she can obtain them.

ALCOHOLISM AND DRUG DEPENDENCE
Self-Evaluation Test

One answer only is required for questions 1–8.

1. Dependence is best defined as:

- **a.** the formation of a habit which strengthens through time;
- **b.** the over-investment of emotion in a pleasurable substance;
- **c.** an intense and prolonged desire for something forbidden;
- **d.** a harmful reliance on one or more chemical substances.

2. The main physiological effect of alcohol is to:

- **a.** stimulate the central nervous system;
- **b.** depress the central nervous system;
- **c.** increase the irritability of muscle fibres;
- **d.** anaesthetise the pripheral nervous system.

3. Increasing tolerance to drugs consists of:

- **a.** the production of antibodies to render them inactive;
- **b.** the elimination of drugs unchanged, without undergoing catabolism;

c. the acquisition of a mental state resistive to their effects;
d. the development of an ability to endure or resist their more harmful effects.

4. Confabulation can be most accurately defined as:
a. filling in memory gaps with detached but inaccurate and fantasised activities;
b. a deliberate attempt to deceive another, concerning one's motives and actions;
c. the unconscious refusal to recognise or accept unwelcome thoughts and wishes;
d. the conscious suppression and control of socially unacceptable fantasies.

5. It is probable that alcoholism is a major problem in Great Britain because:
a. most persons are highly exposed to drinking and can afford alcohol;
b. competitive, highly mobile societies can create extreme psychological stress.
c. cultural patterns encourage a high intake of alcohol
d. mass media advertising programmes feature alcohol as being sophisticated and desirable.
(i) a only
(ii) b,d
(iii) a,b,d
(iv) all of the above.

6. Medical authorities are nearly unanimous in regarding alcoholism as:
a. deviant behaviour;
b. a cultural problem;
c. a treatable disease;
d. a genetic aberration.

7. Which of the following has a great potential for physical dependence:
a. barbiturate;
b. marijuana;
c. amphetamines;
d. cigarettes?

8. Alcoholism could be effectively reduced in this country by:
- **a.** banning the manufacture and sale of alcohol;
- **b.** education encouraging responsible drinking practices;
- **c.** making alcohol a luxury most people can't afford;
- **d.** imposing severe prison sentences on persons suffering from alcoholism.

Assertion and reason

Each of the questions in this section consists of an assertion followed by a reason. Assign to each question one of the five categories (a–e) given in the key below:

KEY
- **a.** The assertion and reason are both true.
  The reason is a correct explanation of the assertion.
- **b.** The assertion and reason are both true.
  The reason is *not* a correct explanation of the assertion.
- **c.** The assertion is true but the reason is false.
- **d.** The assertion is false but the reason is true.
- **e.** The assertion and reasons are both false.

ASSERTION
1. Group therapy is the treatment of choice for the alcoholic patient.

REASON
There is a danger of transferring dependence when drugs are used in the treatment of alcoholism.

ASSERTION
2. Drug-dependent patients are best treated in an authoritarian manner by the nursing staff.

REASON
There is a risk that hospitalisation of drug-dependent patients may foster dependency on the nurses.

ASSERTION
3. The nurse should be closely involved with the drug-dependent patient during the withdrawal period.

REASON
The withdrawal period is an excellent time to begin building a therapeutic relationship with the drug-dependent patient.

ASSERTION
5. Social rehabilitation is an essential part of the successful treatment of drug-dependence.

REASON
Drug-dependent patients who leave treatment centres prematurely almost always relapse.

ASSERTION
6. Nurses may experience difficulty in being objective about alcoholic and drug-dependent patients.

REASON
Alcoholism and drug-dependence are regarded by some as self-imposed states, and as such deserve little sympathy.

True/False items

1. If one drinks only beer, one cannot become alcoholic. (True; False)
2. It is difficult to distinquish between excessive drinking and alcohol-dependence. (True; False)
3. Multiple drug abuse is increasing amongst the young. (True; False)
4. Alcholics will readily admit to their need for help. (True; False)
5. Alcoholism and drug abuse is more likely to occur in persons with poor personality development. (True; False)
6. Alcohol is a drug. (True; False)
7. Society holds similar attitudes to alcohol as it does towards 'soft' drugs. (True; False)
8. There is mounting evidence suggesting that abuse of 'soft' drugs leads to 'hard' drug abuse. (True; False)
9. Abuse of barbiturate drugs frequently follows its legitimate prescription. (True; False)
10. The attitudes of the treatment team towards drug abuse may influence the outcome of the treatment programme. (True; False)

REFERENCES AND FURTHER READING

Cockett, R. (1971), *Drug Abuse and Personality in Young Offenders*, Butterworths.
Cook, T. (1975), *Vagrant Alcoholics*, Routledge & Kegan Paul.
Jellinek, E. M. (1960), *The disease concept of Alcoholism.*
Keller, M. (1960), *New Haven Quarterly Journal of Studies in Alcohol*, **21**, 125.
Keller, M. (1972), On the loss of Control Phenomenon in Alcoholism. *Br. J. Addict.*, **67** (3).
Kessel, N. and Walton, H. (1975), *Alcoholism*, Pelican.
Laurie, P. (1978), *Drugs*, Pelican.
Leech, K. (1974), *A Practical Guide to the Drug Scene*, Sheldon Press.
Mead, J., 'Control yourself – or Enjoy a Drink', *Nursing Mirror* 4.10.74, Vol. 149 No. 14.
Office of Health Economics (1971), *Alcohol and Drug Abuse.*
Robinson, D. (1976), *From Drinking to Alcoholism: a Social Commentary*, John Wiley & Sons.
Royal College of Psychiatrists (1979), *Alcohol and Alcoholism.*
Schofield, M. (1971), *The Strange Case of Pot*, Pelican.
Willis, J. H. (1970), *Drug Dependence*, Faber.

Unit 8

Nursing the Suspicious Patient

INTRODUCTION

Pathological suspicion, in the form of persecutory delusions, ideas of reference and paranoid hostility, may arise in many psychiatric disorders amongst which depression and arteriosclerotic dementia stand out. However, when such symptoms occur in the absence of gross signs of some other disorder it is referred to as a paranoid state of which paranoid schizophrenia, paranoia and paraphrenia are claimed to be variants. Such disorders commonly arise around the age of 30–40 although paraphrenia is particularly common amongst the elderly. Paranoid disorders may occur in acute episodes or run a chronic intractable course. Because of the nature of these disorders some patients represent a serious threat to the safety of others and require treatment in one of the special secure units or hospitals. Most, however, can be treated successfully with modern drug therapy in a conventional psychiatric setting and may benefit from exposure to the social milieu of the hospital.

This unit aims to develop your understanding of the paranoid disorders and to develop your skills in the management of such patients.

It might be helpful to start this unit by reminding ourselves of the point we made in the unit on mental health: this was that abnormal behaviour differs from the normal in degree rather than kind and that its abnormality is largely determined by community norms and the level of tolerance within that community. Many people experience paranoid feelings but are able to maintain some measure of control; these people are not regarded by their peers as abnormal in the pathological sense. Nevertheless they are often brooding, sensitive, secretive people who tend to blame others for their misfortunes and inadequacies and many harbour quite irrational attitudes towards the police, the Department of Health and Social Security or their neighbours etc.

1. Select a patient you have nursed with a paranoid disorder and write a descriptive profile highlighting the main clinical features.

2. What is meant by primary and systematised delusions? Give examples in patients you have nursed.

Delusions of grandiose nature often occur in association with persecutory ideas. The grandiose feelings explain and support, in the mind of the patient, the experience of being watched or plotted against. He comes to believe he must be of great importance to justify such attention. It is not unusual for such patients to believe they are of royal birth, or that they have some divine mission to perform.

The main emotional undercurrents of paranoid reactions are chronic feelings of insecurity and distrust, accompanied by feelings of hostility and low self-esteem. It is to protect himself from such feelings that the patient employs the mental defence mechanism projection. We have also been impressed by the frequency with which depressive feelings seem to accompany or precede upsurges of paranoid feeling. The recognition of such feeling is important if the nurse is to successfully look after such patients.

People suffering from paranoid reaction may benefit from the corrective emotional experience of one–one contact with nursing personnel. Through this relationship they may be helped towards a greater sense of security and trust and helped to increase their feelings of confidence and self-esteem. As a result they may gradually begin to engage in a more open way with others and participate more fully in life. Such relationships take time and are difficult to build. In addition to developing a sensitivity to the patient's needs and feelings the nurse needs to adopt a determined attitude and be reliable, consistent and accepting in her approach. The nurse may often feel she is walking a tightrope in that one inappropriate remark touching on a sensitive area may bring the relationship crashing down; for this reason the nurse should take steps to familiarise herself fully with the background to the patient's illness. In the early stages it is best to avoid being over-friendly and to avoid asking probing questions. Direct discussion of the patient's delusional thinking should also be avoided, as delusional ideas will usually subside and disperse in time and the nurse should support this process by encouraging the patient to apply his thoughts to more neutral topics. Clearly in some instances patients will need to express their fears and anger; here the nurse should listen in a calm accepting way, giving what reassurance she can. She should try to avoid being drawn into an argument about the validity of the patient's feelings and ideas, but if forced to take up a position should always gently try to orientate the patient towards reality.

3. Mrs Grace C., aged 37, has been in hospital four months. She is suffering from a paranoid reaction and is detained in hospital under Section 26 of the Mental Health Act. Grace believes she has been appointed by the Queen to perform some special mission, but that special agents are everywhere trying to prevent her carrying this out. She insists on lining her bed-springs with layers of newspapers which act as a barrier against the radio-active forces that would otherwise enter her body while she was sleeping. She will occasionally make impulsive assaults on people she believes are plotting against her. Grace believes the Queen has a purpose for her in the hospital and therefore accepts the restrictions of hospitalisation.
   a. Grace comes to you and tells you that the patient you have just been talking to can transmit X-rays and that you should avoid looking at her eyes. How might you best respond? Try and be specific.
   b. Maintaining the patient's contact with reality is an important factor in the care of all patients with a psychotic disorder.
      Discuss ways in which you might achieve this objective with this patient.

Aggressive outbursts are fairly common in paranoid disorders but much can be done to prevent them occurring and to minimise the seriousness of such incidents when they do occur. Actions that might aggravate the patient's suspicious feelings and increase tension can be avoided by thoughtful care. Any changes in routine, medication or diet should be carefully explained to the patient before implementation. Inflexible ward rules will increase tension as will forcing the patient to 'join in' before he is ready to mix with others. It is important that a clear policy should be adopted by the treatment team to ensure that their approach to the patient's care is a consistent one. Any restrictions that are to be imposed on the patient should be made clear to him at an early stage. It is often helpful to ask the social worker to advise on and organise the patient's benefits while in hospital as these are a common source of frustration.

Diversional and displacement activities such as craft work, painting, board games and physical recreation are always helpful, to relieve tension and 'damp down' paranoid thinking. They may need to be ward-based initially because of the need for security and supervision. The ward atmosphere is important – it should be relaxed, unthreatening, well-organised, bright and clean, to encourage in the patient a feeling of security and trust. It is our experience that in the early post-admission period it is best to allocate the patient a single room. This helps the patient to develop a sense of security and provides him with a means of taking 'time out' of the ward situation when tensions and persecutory feelings begin to increase.

Good observation is essential to the care of patients with paranoid disorders. Because of the nature of these disorders some patients constitute a serious threat to the safety of others. Many are detained under Section 26 and 65 of the Mental Health Act and the hospital has a responsibility to provide custody as well as therapy. Observation should be as unobtrusive as possible and is best achieved by the nurse participating with the patient in his daily activities, as much as seems appropriate. At all other times it is important for the nurse assigned to the patient to be aware of his whereabouts and of the current policy regarding his management. The nurse should observe for signs of increasing tension, withdrawal, irritability, suspiciousness, guardedness, depression and hallucinatory experience and report any change in behaviour to the senior nurse. The prominence and content of the patient's delusional thinking is a useful guide to progress and management and should also be carefully noted. Positive aspects of the patient's behaviour should also be looked for: relaxation, trust, rational thinking and participation with others are all indicators that progress is being made.

4. Miss J., aged 65, has always been a rather seclusive and eccentric person. Recently she has taken to barricading herself in her house, conversing with callers and paying tradesmen through the letterbox. She believes that people in the neighbourhood are draining her 'life forces' through their radios, she is admitted to your unit with a diagnosis of paraphrenia. She is watchful, tense and suspicious and at times appears to respond to auditory hallucinations.

   i. Outline the main points of the nursing care of this patient.
   ii. Why would it be therapeutically undesirable to allow this lady to remain socially isolated following discharge.
   iii. Deafness is often associated with late paraphrenia. Explain how this may give rise to paranoid reactions.

5. Mr Tony D., aged 36, has been in hospital for two months. He is a married man, now separated, and currently unemployed. He is described as a withdrawn and reticent man who has always felt insecure and inadequate in his relationship with others and particularly with women. His persecutory feelings centre around a delusion concerning his wife's fidelity. Mrs D. reported that Tony had begun to follow her everywhere and would search her handbag and clothing when she came home for evidence of her involvement with other men. He began to believe that people passing in the street were watching the house waiting for him to leave; he became convinced that his wife's lovers were trying to poison him. Admission followed an incident in which he impulsively assaulted his next-door neighbour, accusing him of trying to emasculate him with an insecticide spray. Tony now appears more relaxed and is thinking on a more rational level. He seems less guarded and is beginning to participate in a more open way with others, particularly the staff.

At a treatment team conference it is suggested that it might be time to consider discharge. What suggestions might you make about his follow-up care?

THE SUSPICIOUS PATIENT

Self-Evaluation Test

1. David A., angrily accuses you of trying to poison him when you offer him his medication. This is an example of . . .

Select the best response from the list below:

a. projection;
b. displacement;
c. rationalization;
d. sublimation.

2. A patient with paranoid feelings confides to you 'they are out to get me. Even the Doctor is in league with them'.

Select the best response from the list below:

a. I can understand how you feel, but it doesn't seem to me that this is so; you will be quite safe here;
b. you are allowing your imagination to run away with you;
c. yes, and the sooner the better; we might get some peace then;
d. you feel that way because you are ill.

3. The pre-illness personality of the paranoid patient is often characterised by:

a. fussy, orderly, meticulous, conscientious behaviour;
b. impulsive, mischievous, unfeeling, anti-social behaviour;
c. brooding, sensitive, secretive, distrustful behaviour;
d. timid, anxious, inadequate, withdrawn behaviour.

4. Mrs J., informs you on your first day on the ward that she owns the hospital and pays your wages. This is an example of . . .
Select the best response from the list below:

a. passivity feelings;
b. delusions of unworthiness;
c. delusions of grandeur;
d. delusions of persecution;
e. delusions of poverty.

5. Select from the list below the best response to Mrs J's statement:

a. I'm so hard up this month do you think you could give me an advance;
b. you feel that way because you are ill;
c. could you tell me a little about the daily routine on this ward, Mrs J;
d. you just imagine that you do; the Health Authority pays our wages.

6. Select from the list below behaviour that would indicate that progress towards stability and health is being made:

a. participation with others;
b. rational thinking;
c. assertiveness;
d. trust;
e. relaxation.
(i) b,c,d,e;
(ii) c,d,e;
(iii) a,b,d,e;
(iv) all of the above.

Assertion and reason

Each of the questions in this section consist of an assertion followed by a reason. Assign to each question one of the five categories (a–e) given in the key below:

KEY
a. The assertion and reason are both true.
The reason is a correct explanation of the assertion.
b. The assertion and reason are both true.
The reason is *not* a correct explanation of the assertion.

c. The assertion is true but the reason is false.
d. The assertion is false but the reason is true.
e. The assertion and reason are both false.

ASSERTION
1. Delusions of grandeur are common in paranoid states.

REASON
They help explain in the minds of the patient why he should be singled out for attention and persecution.

ASSERTION
2- Good observation is an essential element in the care of patients suffering from paranoid states.

REASON
The risk of suicide is high.

ASSERTION
3. Social isolation is an important causative factor in paraphrenia.

REASON
The individual is unable to test the reality of his experiences and is not constrained by group conformity.

ASSERTION
4. Diversional activities are helpful in the care of suspicious patients.

REASON
Tension is relieved and delusional thinking damped down.

ASSERTION
5. Ideas of reference are delusions in which the patient feels he is being influenced and controlled by unseen forces.

REASON
The paranoid person is very sensitive to his environment and frequently misinterprets it as being hostile to him.

ASSERTION
6. Inconsistent care may provoke aggressive outbursts.

REASON
Feelings of distrust and insecurity are exacerbated.

ASSERTION

7. A bright, cheerful, friendly approach is the best way of facilitating a relationship with paranoid patients.

REASON

It fosters a sense of security and trust.

True/False Items

1. Depressive moods often accompany an increase in paranoid thinking. (True; False)
2. Paraphrenia is most common amongst the elderly. (True; False)
3. Delusional ideas can usually be dispersed by rational argument. (True; False)
4. Systematised delusions are delusional ideas; ideas linked by a central theme. (True; Falsee)
5. Hallucinations may occur in severe paranoid states. (True; False)
6. Group activities should be positively encouraged from the start of treatment. (True; False)

REFERENCES AND FURTHER READING

Batchelor, I., (1968), *Henderson and Gillespie's Textbook of Psychiatry*, Oxford University Press.
Crowcroft, A. (1967), *The Psychotic*, Pelican.
Mereness, D. (1978), *Essentials of Psychiatric Nursing*, Mosby.
Storr, A. (1968), *Human Aggression*, Penguin.

Unit 9

Nursing the Withdrawn Patient

INTRODUCTION

Many people have a tendency to escape into social withdrawal when the frustrations and pressures of life become too demanding. In this way they 'insulate' themselves against the world and indulge in compensatory day-dreams and fantasy. Provided withdrawal is not used excessively it can be a helpful way of softening the impact of stress.

Behaviour characterised by pathological withdrawal is, however, fairly common in psychiatric hospitals. The term 'withdrawal' is used both in the social sense to mean a person who seeks to isolate themselves from others and in the psychological sense to mean that the person's appreciation of, and contact with, reality is limited. Withdrawal is the central feature of a serious psychotic illness called schizophrenia.

Much has been achieved in recent years in the treatment and management of this disorder and although it continues to produce chronic disability the outlook for most is much brighter. The reason for this therapeutic optimism has been the concurrent developments in drug therapy and social psychiatry over the last thirty years.

This unit aims to develop your skill in the management of the withdrawn patient and to increase your understanding of the role of the nurse in the rehabilitation and community support of such patients. We have also included in this unit a section on institutionalisation. It is appropriate to explore this topic here because of the vulnerability to institutionalisation of patients with schizophrenia. It should be remembered, however, that any patient requiring long-term care, including the elderly, is at risk. Schizophrenia is a serious and disabling psychotic illness which is found throughout the world and affects 0.85 per cent of the population of the U.K., Currently around 35,000 people are in hospital suffering from this illness and many others are being supported by community-care teams in their own homes, in group homes, and in hostel accommodation. A schizophrenic illness may occur at any age but it is most common amongst young adults. The onset may be insidious over a number of years with increasing withdrawal, poverty of thought, inertia and self-neglect as the prominent features; or acute with excitability, incoherent speech, bizarre behaviour, delusions and hallucinations prominent.

1. Schizophrenia has a severe and disruptive effect on many aspect of the personality. Using the headings below, describe the various signs and symptoms which may be present.

Disorder of thought.
Disorder of emotions.
Disorder of volition.
Disorder of perception.
Disorder of behaviour.

2. Write a descriptive profile of a patient suffering from a schizophrenic illness whom you have nursed.

3. The cause of schizophrenia remains unknown. Briefly outline the theories of causation listed below:

Genetic theory.
Neurochemical theory.
Ego psychology theory.
Perceptual filter theory.
Family interaction theory.

The prognosis in schizophrenia is variable. Some illnesses run a chronic course with a progressive deterioration of the patient's social functioning. This has given rise to the 'social drift' phenomenon which is characterised by the medically unsupported schizophrenic slowly descending the social ladder to eventually live a vagrant-like existence in squalid urban surroundings. Remissions have sometimes been reported in middle age. Happily other patients with the illness respond well to treatment, and remain stable and relatively well-adjusted socially for long periods. Factors which appear to indicate a good prognosis are acute onset, emotional responsiveness, the absence of a family history of the illness, a previously well integrated personality, late onset, clear precipitating factors and good average intelligence.

The social atmosphere of the ward and hospital in which the patient is being treated is an important factor influencing the course of the illness. There is always the danger that once hospitalised the patient may have imposed on him a role which is essentially a passive and submissive one. There may be little opportunity to make decisions or to exercise any responsibility for his own life or the lives of others, and long periods of the day may be spent in inactivity and isolation. Such situations must be avoided as they tend to reinforce and exacerbate behaviour patterns characteristic of the illness such as withdrawal and inertia. Many studies for example, Wing, 1968 have emphasised the therapeutic benefits to the schizophrenic of appropriate social and occupational stimulus. Conversely, it is also true that intense and demanding social stimulus may cause an increase in the florid symptoms of the illness. For example, some confrontation at work or at home may precipitate excitable bizarre behaviour, incoherent speech and delusional or hallucinatory experience, creating the typical pre-admission crisis. Similar reactions may occur on admission to hospital following transfer to another ward, following a change of ward staff or on excursions outside hospital. There is, therefore, an optimum level of stimulus that must be found to achieve maximum therapeutic benefit from the treatment programme. During the acute phase the patient should be nursed in a calm, quiet, restful atmosphere. Activities should be relaxing and diversional with the nurse providing supportive care of an emotional and physical nature. Following the acute phase the programme can be 'geared up' but should be consistent, predictable and rehabilitative, but not too intense.

A well-structured day is most important in the therapeutic care and rehabilitation of people with schizophrenia. It should approximate life in the community at large and should reflect an appreciation of the needs of individual patients. Healthy social habits such as work habits, good personal hygiene and appearance, social involvement with others, are often lost in this illness. It is therefore essential that the daily programme ensures the maintenance and reinforcement of such habits. Activities should be group-centred wherever possible. The group should provide support and encouragement, help the individual develop social skills and confidence, counter isolation and withdrawal and encourage clear rational thinking. In addition, exposures to subtle group pressures to conform to group norms may help normalise behaviour and change unhelpful attitudes. There are many activities that may be organised on a group basis: industrial therapy in a workshop atmosphere, a horticulture group, clerical group, domestic management retraining group, play-reading and musical-appreciation groups, physical-fitness group, socio-drama group, art and craft groups. Discussion group, resocialization/re-activation groups are examples of groups which may help alleviate symptoms and facilitate rehabilitation.

4. Discuss the organisation and the relevance of any three of the group activities mentioned in the rehabilitation of patients with schizophrenia whom you have nursed.

The relationship the nurse is able to form with the schizophrenic patient is a key factor in social therapy. Establishing such a relationship can, however, be a difficult and demanding experience. Often the lack of emotional and verbal responsiveness, or the irrationality or inconsequential nature of the patient's conversation, make it difficult to feel any real contact has been made. It is not unusual for nurses in such situations to feel rejected or inadequate and to avoid contact with such patients seeking out the more responsive and socially rewarding patients in their care. It should be kept in mind that the patient's unresponsiveness and irrational behaviour is an attempt to cope with frightening and confusing experiences. Despite the deceptively flattened affect and inertia of many schizophrenics the arousal level is often high and withdrawal offers them some sanctuary. The withdrawn patient will usually respond in time to sensitive, thoughtful and persistent social contact with the nurse. The nurse should try to foster a sense of security and confidence in her patients and give positive encouragement to any appropriate social response, however small.

5. Describe how you have used/could use a behavioural approach to encourage more adaptive behaviour in schizophrenic patients whom you have nursed.

It is largely through his interaction with the nurse that the patient is able to test reality. That is, he is able to determine which of his experiences have a firm basis in the real world and which are distortions. For this reason the nurse should always avoid the temptation to give support to a patient's delusional thinking, and should always gently direct the patient's thoughts towards reality and clear rational thinking.

Hallucinations which are usually of a auditory nature may be distressing. Sometimes patients will behave in impulsive ways, for example injuring themselves in response to hallucinatory voices. Careful observation should therefore be maintained. Actively hallucinating patients need considerable reassurance and supervision, and simple diversional activity may be helpful.

You will have noticed that patients with this illness often have difficulty in organising and maintaining their thought-flow. For this reason it is helpful if the nurse keeps her conversation with such patients simple and matter of fact. She should avoid deep-searching or demanding discussions, as this will only add to the patient's perplexity and confusion.

The nurse should play particular attention to non-verbal signals, the emotional tone and symbolism in the patient's conversation, as often such factors may convey meaning to what is being expressed unintelligibly.

Participation with the patient in his day-to-day activities is an important principle of care. It provides the opportunity for observation and assessment of the patient's social functioning – how well he copes with work, his hygiene and appearance, social contact with others, domestic responsibilities, leisure time etc. It also provides the opportunity for interaction between the nurse and the patient to take place in an informal, personalised atmosphere and for the nurse to give encouragement and support. In addition, working closely with the patient the nurse is able to serve as a role model with whom the patient can identify.

6. Comment on how you have used/may be able to use the process of identification to encourage healthy behaviour patterns in patients with schizophrenia whom you have nursed.

One problem the nurse will experience constantly is how to motivate her patients. She will need to overcome the inertia and resistiveness that is a common feature of the illness if her patients are to benefit fully from the therapeutic programme. We have already commented on how the behavioural approach and the process of identification may help in this task. It is most important that the patient should be adequately informed of the reasons for the nurse's requests and directions. He should know why various aspects of his care and treatment programme are important to him and how well he is performing. The activity programme must be sufficiently interesting and satisfying to encourage attendance and participation. Incentives in the form of payments, a sense of accomplishment, companionship, a pleasant working environment etc., are essential. In addition the nurse will need to adopt a determined and persuasive approach if she is to be successful in gaining the patient's co-operation. Although many patients will require continued prompting and supervision the nurse must always be on the look-out for the opportunity to encourage initiative and self-reliance and be aware of indications that the patient is ready to assume more personal responsibility for his day-to-day life.

As in any community, limits on behaviour must be set, and the nurse must be prepared to exert more control and direction if the patient's behaviour deviates too far. However, she should try not to be too inflexible in her implementation of the care programme and should remember that patients may have very different standards, values and interests from her own, and these must be respected.

7. Some patients with this illness have a very fragmented and distorted sense of their own identity. This sometimes leads them to adopt the identity of fellow-patients or staff, to talk in the third person or to feel that their thoughts and actions affect, in an adverse way, the helped well-being of others. Suggest ways in which you have helped/may be able to help patients develop and retain a sense of self-identity.

8. Miss Sheila D., aged 21, has been a patient on your ward for about three weeks and was admitted under Section 25 of the Mental Health Act. She is described as a quiet, sensitive girl who has grown up in the shadow of her rather dominating and over-protective mother. Sheila notably lacks the assurance and confidence you would expect in a girl her age, and has little idea of the practicalities of day-to-day life. She is quite a bright girl but has only been able to hold jobs for short periods owing to her lack of social poise. She was admitted to hospital in an agitated and excited state. She said that she was changing and that her face was made of china clay. She complained of hearing men's voices inside her head, making sexual suggestions. Shortly after admission Sheila assaulted one of the male patients on the unit, claiming that it was his voice in her brain. Sheila is now more composed but tends to spend long periods sitting by herself twisting strands of hair, preoccupied with her thoughts. She shows little spontaneous interest in herself or the activities of the unit, and her conversation continues to show traces of confused delusional thinking.

Work out a programme of activities to meet the needs of this patient, indicating what your responsibilities and involvement might be.

INSTITUTIONALIZATION

In addition to the damaging effects of the illness on the patient's personality and social functioning he may be further disabled by a process called institutionalization. Institutionalization is brought about by elements in the patient's social environment which combine to stifle independence, individuality and personal growth. Institutionalized patients lose self-reliance and confidence, are unable to make decisions and carry out many of the basic activities of day-to-day life. They lose the desire to pursue normal social goals such as employment, a home and a partner outside the institution. Many become submissive and lose all individuality and interest.

Despite the upgrading of wards to create a more attractive and homely living environment, and despite the influence of social psychiatry on attitudes and organisation, there is little room for complacency. Inflexible, rigid ward routines persist that provide little opportunity for the expression of personal initiative and responsibility, or for decision-making to take place. Activities are often not rehabilitative and lack interest and variety. Staff attitudes are often characterised by benign authoritarianism and therapeutic pessimism. Their social expectations of patients are also often unhelpfully low. Contact with the community is for many often infrequent, despite the open doors and the emphasis given to community involvement. Nor should we confine our thinking to hospital care. Institutionalisation may occur in patients living in community hostels, or at home, if the fabric of their daily lives and the attitudes of those involved with them do not allow and encourage personal development. Patients with schizophrenia are particularly vulnerable to the institutionalising effect of the social factors described. They have often not built up strong ties with the community, prior to their illness, through marriage, work and leisure interests. They may have never been concerned with decision-making or self-assertion, and their involvement with others may have been minimal. Such people very quickly become dependent on institutional support.

9. Barton (1959) has described institutionalization in terms of a clinical syndrome which he called institutional neurosis.

Write a descriptive profile of a patient you have nursed suffering from institutional neurosis.

10. Below is a list of the causative factors in institutional neurosis. Write a brief account of each of those, showing how they arise both in the hospital and community setting; suggest ways in which they may be prevented.

Loss of contact with the ouside world.

Enforced idleness.
Brutality, bossiness and teasing.
Loss of personal friends, possessions and events.
Demoralising ward atmosphere.
Loss of prospects in the community.
Excessive use of tranquillisers and sedatives.

Awareness of these factors has led to new concepts on the care of the long-stay patient. Many traditional long-stay wards have become much more like hostels providing varying levels of staff supervision.

The atmosphere is homely and comfortable. Full use is made of available single accommodation and the dormitory areas are organised to allow the maximum of privacy and to encourage personalisation of the bed space. Patients are referred to as residents, and staff have largely abandoned their clinical role along with their uniforms in favour of the role of 'instructor'. Much more is done with the patient rather than to the patient and relationships become more personalised. Such wards are fully equipped with washing and cooking facilities to encourage independence. A weekly community meeting involves the residents in making decisions that affect their lives and the lives of others. At such meetings domestic matters are discussed, leisure activities planned and individual problems and progress discussed. This helps develop a sense of community and encourages healthy norms and goals amongst the resident group. They become aware that initiative, independence, social responsiveness, good hygiene and work attendance bring tangible rewards such as more pocket money, a room of their own, a transfer to a better ward, a more interesting work situation, a place in a group home, etc. Every effort is made to normalise the environment: there are no medicine rounds, many receive long-acting depot drugs, others are encouraged to collect their medication or look after it themselves. Any necessary treatments are carried out in the out-patients department, and residents who need to see a doctor make an appointment to see him in his consulting room as they would in the community. All patients work at some useful 'paid' occupation. Many work in the hospital workshop doing contract work for outside industry. Others work in the carpentry or clerical sections of the occupational therapy department and some as catering or domestic assistants within the hospital. The emphasis is on making the work situation as realistic as possible. Residents are expected to arrive on time, be productive, report sick, take holidays, work co-operatively with others and receive a wage for their efforts in the usual way. In addition to their work placement other rehabilitative activities, e.g. domestic management will form part of their daily programme.

In these days of high unemployment it is perhaps unrealistic to expect many patients to compete in the labour market. The constructive and satisfying use of leisure is therefore of great importance in the rehabilitation programme. Many people find it difficult to use unstructured time and need assistance to achieve this. Individual or small-group activities, if possible initiated and planned by the patients themselves, are preferable to staff-organised 'institutional' activities. Leisure activities should be community-orientated as much as possible, with regular visits to the shops, local pub, cinemas, swimming baths, etc.

11. Under the guidance of your charge nurse organise a social excursion for a *small* group of patients, e.g. shopping expedition, picnic, visit to a local pub for a drink and a game of darts.

- **i.** Select one patient from your group; write a brief clinical synopsis and comment on his behaviour during the activity.
- **ii.** How may this and similar activities be of benefit to the patients in your group?

12. Under the guidance of your charge nurse organise a hospital-based social evening for a group of patients. You should try and involve your patients in planning for and organising the event; you may like to involve relatives or a local community organisation.

- **i.** Select one patient from your group; write a brief clinical synopsis and comment on their behaviour during the evening.
- **ii.** How may this and similar activities be of benefit to patients in your group?

As we have already outlined in this unit chronic disability often takes the form of an amalgam of institutionalism and the more persistent features of the primary illness. Thus the behaviour of many patients who have been hospitalised for any length of time is characterised by loss of initiative, social withdrawal, poor hygiene, dress and work habits. Conversational defects such as poverty of speech, delusional speech or 'crazy talk' are usually present and behaviour may take an aggressive, excitable, incongruous, negativistic or manneristic form.

Many of these problems can be overcome or reduced by the nursing team judiciously and consistently using a reward system to develop and reinforce healthy adaptive behaviour and by becoming more conscious of the importance of not reinforcing abnormal behaviour, e.g. rewarding normal speech and ignoring delusional or bizarre speech. There is a tendency for nurses to pay attention to the more deviant aspects of patients' behaviour and thus unwittingly reinforce and perpetuate such behaviour, and less attention to the healthy aspects of patients' behaviour which could be developed.

Before reading on, you may find it helpful to return again to the unit on mental health where the theories that support the behavioural approach to care and treatment are outlined.

Tokens which have an exchange value have been used with some success as reinforcers to encourage more adaptive behaviour in behavioural regimes. Social rewards in the form of praise – 'well done', 'that's great', and the increased attention of the staff – sitting next to the patient, chatting sociably to him – are also potent reinforcers. Not all patients, of course, find increased attention rewarding; it is therefore important that the staff make the contact pleasurable for the patient or find other reinforcers.

13. Suggest items other than those mentioned that might have value as reinforcers.

To be effective a reinforcer must be given consistently, immediately after the behaviour has occurred, and if social reinforcers are being used they must be expressed genuinely and with enthusiasm. Reinforcement should always be accompanied with feedback so that the association between the reward and the behaviour can be made, e.g., 'that's terrific, John, you really look smart'.

As we have said, many patients lack motivation and initiative and the nurse may have to initiate the desired behaviour in the early stages of treatment by prompting the patient. Sometimes this is the essence of the problem in that the patient is really quite capable of carrying out the task but lacks the initiative to start or to see it through. Staff should try to stand back as often as possible and let their patients take decisions and experience the consequences of their own behaviour. Any show of initiative should be reinforced, and where prompting is required it should be phased out as quickly as possible. Using indirect prompts, 'Isn't it time you went for lunch, collected your tablets?' etc, and then as the patient becomes more self-reliant, just non-verbal cues, such as a glance at the clock, will help rekindle initiative.

In trying to develop new behaviour staff must give the patient clear, simple instructions; often modelling the desired behaviour yourself is a more effective way of conveying what is required, particuarly in work or social situations. The nurse–patient relationship is particularly important here as a patient will imitate more readily a nurse he likes. Sometimes the target behaviour is too difficult for the patient to reach in one step, and can best be achieved in small stages. Building up behaviour in this way is called shaping. The nurse successively reinforces behaviour that approximates to the target behaviour. For example a patient who has not shaved himself for years may be reinforced successively first for holding the shaving brush, then for soaping his face partially, then totally, then for holding the razor correctly and so on until the complete sequence has been achieved. As with all learning continued practice is important in consolidating behaviour.

Undesirable behaviour can be reduced or eliminated in a number of ways. One approach is to consistently reinforce incompatible behaviour, e.g. rewarding a manneristic patient for adopting acceptable movements and posture. Another approach is to try and eliminate behaviour through the process called extinction. In extinction the reduction and disappearance of some undesirable aspect of behaviour depends on the identification and removal of the source of reinforcement. Behaviour that is not reinforced will cease. If for example the bizarre speech of a patient attracts amused attention from the staff, thus reinforcing it, ignoring such behaviour in a fairly obvious way – walking away, looking bored and uninterested etc, will lead eventually to its extinction. One problem with this approach is that of maintaining consistency, as people other than the nursing team may reinforce the undesirable behaviour. Some forms of deviant behaviour are difficult to ignore because of their disruptive or dangerous nature.

A further approach to this problem of reducing undesirable behaviour is the use of punishment in the form of reprimands, restriction to the ward, reduction of cigarette ration, etc., in response to the occurrence of undesirable behaviour. It is likely that such an approach will only serve to suppress behaviour rather than eliminate it, and to be successful this must be combined with feedback and positive reinforcement of acceptable behaviour patterns. A procedure known as 'time out' has been successfully used to reduce some forms of disruptive and destructive behaviour such as indecent behaviour, shouting and swearing, deliberate provocation of others, smashing up, etc. When such episodes occur the patient should be removed promptly to a single room without fuss and without explanation. The period of isolation should be of short duration, the patient being allowed to circulate freely again as soon as his behaviour becomes acceptable. Thus the patient is removed from the potential or actual positive reinforcers of the abnormal behaviour and begins to behave in the desired way to avoid punishment, i.e. negative reinforcement.

You may find it helpful at this point to refer to the section on the attention-seeking patient where the disadvantages of using punishment to change behaviour are outlined.

14. Mr William L., aged 43, has been in hospital almost continuously for the past 20 years. He suffers from schizophrenia and his behaviour is characterised by the residual features of this disorder and by the adverse effects of institutional life. He needs prompting with washing, bathing collecting his medicines, attending OT and recreational functions. His dress has a careless dishevelled appearance, his washing and shaving habits are not very thorough, and he almost always forgets to comb his hair and brush his teeth. His speech is often bizarre and delusional and he has frequent episodes of shouting and swearing if he doesn't get his own way. William attends the carpentry section of the OT but is reported to be incapable of all but simple asks and not very productive. William is something of a hospital character because of his humorous, inventive speech. He likes all the attention he gets and the numerous cigarettes and cups of tea he obtains for his 'performances'.

Describe how the nursing team might employ a behavioural approach to try and modify this patient's behaviour.

15. Mrs Janet T., aged 46, has been more or less permanently hospitalised for the past 14 years. She is now divorced from her husband and has little contact with her married daughter who lives in the area. The symptoms of her illness now appear minimal and the overall impression is of an apathetic, dependent, overweight lady. She lacks a great deal of motivation and confidence and takes little responsibility for the events of her day-to-day life. Staff have to supervise Janet's hygiene, appearance and work attendance and help her care for her belongings. She shows little interest in the outside world and shows no ambition to leave the hospital. She works daily in the hospital sewing room but staff report that her lack of confidence, poor concentration and effort reduce her contribution to a minimum. Janet has a habit of adopting a stooped posture, and frequently rocks when sitting down.

At a staff meeting of the ward treatment team it is decided that Janet would be a good subject for rehabilitation. Work out a programme of activities you think would help this patient, indicating what your involvement and responsibilities might be.

TIME	ACTIVITY	RESPONSIBILITY & INVOLVEMENT
7.00 a.m. 9.00 a.m.		
9.00 a.m. 12.00		
12.00 2.00 p.m.		
2.00 p.m. 5.00 p.m.		
5.00 p.m. 7.00 p.m.		
7.00 p.m. 10.00 p.m.		

COMMUNITY CARE

The availability of effective treatment for schizophrenia, coupled with more tolerant and informed social attitudes, has meant that many more patients with this illness are now being cared for outside hospital. The principles of care we have been discussing in relation to the hospitalised patient apply equally to the patient being treated in the community. However, helping the patient in the community to regain some measure of stablity and improve his social functioning is clearly a more difficult proposition than in hospital because of the problem of controlling the social relationships and the environment to which the patient is exposed. For example isolation and inactivity may occur and be just as damaging in the community, or the emotional atmosphere at home may not be conducive to the patient's continued stability. A great deal of time may be spent by the nurse providing support and developing helpful attitudes within the family. It should be remembered that the withdrawn patient may place quite a burden on the family, and if we are to avoid a backlash against the trend towards community care we must ensure that our community services are both reliable and effective.

Re-establishing the patient in the community after a period of hospitalisation may present many problems. One problem is the provision of suitable accommodation. People in hospital very quickly lose their foothold in the community. Families are often reluctant to take the patient back, particularly if there have been problems coping with disturbed behaviour in the past. Others have become accustomed to living their lives without the patient; his position in the family may have become redundant, so that if he does return home a great deal of readjustment is necessary.

As we have indicated it is sometimes therapeutically undesirable for the patient to return to live with his family where the unhealthy emotional atmosphere and abnormal pattern of communication may encourage the reappearance of abnormal behaviour. One possibility is the community hostel. Here the patient can live as a member of a small group, in a supportive atmosphere, with the rights and responsibilities of an ordinary citizen, and must face up to day-to-day challenges of life in the community. It is important that the hostel develops a social organisation that encourages personal growth and independence, and does not foster institutionalism.

16. A most helpful development in recent years has been the establishment of group homes. These are ordinary family houses in new or established residential areas which allow patients to live in small family groups with a minimum of supervision. Using the following headings discuss some of the difficulties that might arise in setting up a group home:

Selection of patients.
Preparation of patients.
The quality of life before and after discharge.

Professional supervision.
The local community.

Work is an important factor in the rehabilitation and continued stability of the patient. It gives a structure to life, and helps develop and maintain a sense of self-esteem, confidence and independence. Work brings the patient into contact with others, and from this contact personal relationships may grow. After a schizophrenic illness patients sometimes experience residual disabilities, are unable to return to their previous employment and require less demanding occupations. For some continued attendance at the hospital OT group or industrial therapy unit may be helpful. A few may be able to attend an industrial rehabilitation unit where employment potential and limitations may be assessed, and some may be taught new skills at government training centres. A number of patients with continuing disabilities will be unable to compete in the employment market and require sheltered employment in local authority workshops. It is most important that community workers are able to establish good relationships with local industry, and that workers in the field of occupational health should have an informed appreciation of the problems of the mentally ill.

Leisure activities and social relationships are important to us all. It is partly through our involvement in various pursuits and with friends that we are able to satisfy many of our social needs and find some measure of satisfaction and fulfilment in our lives. The schizophrenic often has difficulty establishing social relationships and pursuing an active social life. The patient should be encouraged to take part in community activities, particularly those where there is an accent on participation and where new members are welcomed and involved. Sports clubs, over-18 clubs, groups affiliated to local churches, rambling clubs, darts teams are some examples.

In some areas community day centres and evening groups have been set up to provide social facilities, continued support and rehabilitation and advice to discharged patients and others. These centres provide a very valuable service helping to combat loneliness, boredom, morbid introspection, self-pity, and help improve independence, confidence and social functioning through their activity programme. Some centres provide workshop facilities where commercial projects have been initiated and most day centres are able to provide a meal.

17. Imagine you have been given the responsibility of organising an activity programme for the twenty members of your local day centre. Outline your programme for a typical day.

18. Mr David C., aged 28, suffers from schizophrenia. This is his third spell in hospital and he has been a patient on your unit for the past four months. Although David's behaviour is still somewhat withdrawn, preoccupied and incongruous he has made good progress since admission and is now working reliably with the OT gardening group and is maintaining a reasonable level of social functioning. It has been decided to refer David to the community team pending discharge to his parents' home. David's parents are somewhat reluctant at this stage to take him home as they have had problems coping with his 'disturbed' behaviour in the past. They complain that he shuts himself in his room, neglects himself and idles away his time. They say that David swears at them and has on occasions been violent when they 'get on to him about his laziness'. They are afraid to go out and leave David by himself and say that their friends no longer call because of his behaviour. Mr C. senior is a vigorous man with a dominant personality. He is irritated by David's apathetic approach to life and frequently compares David with his more outgoing and successful older brother. Mrs C. tends to be a rather passive and possessive person who sees David as a quiet home-loving boy who needs looking after.

What are the needs of the patient and his family? Develop a community care programme to meet these needs.

NURSING THE WITHDRAWN PATIENT

Self-Evaluation test

1. Acute schizophrenia is characterised by . . .

Select the most appropriate response from the list below:

a. apathetic, helpless, submissive behaviour;
b. confident, aggressive, overactive behaviour;
c. excitable, bizarre, withdrawn beaviour;
d. timid, anxious, withdrawn behaviour.

2. Thought disorder in schizophrenia is characcterised by . . .

Select the *two* most appropriate responses from the list below:

a. flight of ideas;
b. thought blocking;
c. perseveration;
d. tangental thinking.

3. Emotional responses in schizophrenia are often described as . . .
Select the most appropriate response from the list below:

a. labile;
b. euphoric;
c. melancholic;
d. flattened.

4. Hallucinations are examples of a disorder of . . .
Select the most appropriate response from the list below:

a. affect;
b. memory;
c. volition;
d. perception.

5. Nurse D. found that by working enthusiastically alongside her patients in the OT department work performance improved. This is an example of . . .

a. identification;
b. displacement;
c. operant conditioning;
d. compliance.

6. Group social activities are helpful in the care of schizophrenic patients. This is because . . .
Select the best response from the list below:

a. control and supervision is easier;
b. they counter isolation and withdrawal;
c. they encourage clear, rational thinking;
d. they provide support and encouragement;
e. problems are explored and insight gained.
(i) a, b, c;
(ii) b, c, d;
(iii) d, e;
(iv) all the above.

7. Apathy, submissiveness, inertia, loss of interest and individuality are features of . . .
Select the best response from the list below:

a. endogenous depression;

b. dementia;
c. schizophrenia;
d. institutionalisation.

8. Which *two* of the following activities would you consider *most* helpful to the schizophrenic:

a. needlework;
b. reading a magazine;
c. playing monopoly;
d. attending a social/dance;
e. going for a walk.

Assertion and reason

Each of the questions in this section consist of an assertion followed by a reason. Assign to each question one of the five categories (a–e) given in the key below:

KEY

a. The assertion and reason are both true.
The reason is a correct explanation of the assertion.
b. The assertion and reason are both true.
The reason is *not* a correct explanation of the assertion.
c. The assertion is true but the reason is false.
d. The assertion is false but the reason is true.
e. The assertion and reason are both false.

ASSERTION

1. Social stimulus which becomes intense and demanding may precipitate acute schizophrenic behaviour in vulnerable individuals.

REASON

The brain cannot effectively 'filter out' stimulus, and becomes overloaded.

ASSERTION

2. Nurses must be firm and use their authority to ensure patients with schizophrenia use their time constructively.

REASON

Laziness is a characteristic of people with schizophrenia.

ASSERTION

3. A well-structured day is an important element in the care of people with schizophrenia.

REASON

Healthy social habits are lost in this illness if the day-to-day activities are not organised and supervised.

ASSERTION

4. The nurse–patient relationship is an important element in social therapy.

REASON

The patient's contact with reality is supported and maintained.

ASSERTION

5. It is not always advisable to discharge the schizophrenic patient to live at home.

REASON

The emotional atmosphere and family attitudes may not be conducive to continued stability.

ASSERTION

6. Patients with schizophrenia often have a confused sense of self-identity.

REASON

Disorientation is a common feature of this illness.

ASSERTION

7. Wards providing accommodation for long-stay patients should be run like hostels.

REASON

A traditionally run ward stifles personal development and fosters dependency.

ASSERTION

8. The intellectual stimulus of an involved discussion is a helpful activity for people with schizophrenia.

REASON

People with this illness have difficulty organising and maintaining their thought flow.

True/False items

1. Group homes are communities where group activities are a central feature of day-to-day life. (True; False)
2. Social drift in schizophrenic illness implies the person is unable to maintain his social position and relationships and gravitates to a poorer quality of life. (True; False)
3. Schizophrenia usually appears in young adulthood. (True; False)
4. The 'double bind' theory is an attempt to explain schizophrenia in terms of a biochemical disorder. (True; False)
5. Visual hallucinations are a common feature of schizophrenia. (True; False)
6. Lack of verbal and emotional responsiveness in schizophrenia makes establishing a nurse–patient relationship difficult. (True; False)

REFERENCES AND FURTHER READING

Barton, R. (1976). *Institutional Neurosis*, Wright.
Butler, R. (1978), *Behaviour and Rehabilitation*, Wright.
Cameron, J. (1958), *Chronic Schizophrenia*, Tavistock.
Clarke, D. (1974), *Social Therapy*, Pelican.
Crowcroft, A. (1967), *The Psychotic*, Pelican.
Jones, M. (1968), *Beyond the Therapeutic Community*, Yale U.P.
Mitchell, A. (1975), *Schizophrenia – What it Means*, Teach Yourself Books.
Priest, R. (1977), *Insanity*, MacDonald Evans.
Wilder, J. (1978), *An Aid to Community Care* Psychiatric Rehab. Assoc.
Wing, J. (1970), *Institutionalism and Schizophrenia*, C.U.P.

Unit 10

Problems Relating to Sexual Activity

INTRODUCTION

Probably the most sensitive area of human relationships is that which involves sexual behaviour. Many people are extremely reluctant to discuss the problems they encounter.

Similarly, nurses often prefer to avoid the subject when patients approach them for advice, or they may lack sufficient expertise to be of real assistance to the patient.

Obviously the nurse's personal attitude both towards acceptable and deviant sexual activity will greatly influence the way he/she will react when approached for counselling. It probably takes a great deal of courage for most patients to ask for advice. An insensitive or critical response by the nurse could be disastrous and may well prevent further effective counselling.

The aims of this unit are to discuss four different age-groups, namely adolescence, young adulthood, middle age and old age, and to consider the common problems relating to sexual behaviour in those groups in order that nurses may be better able to give counsel and advice. In addition, modern forms of sex therapy will be discussed briefly.

It is not intended to discuss in detail the different types of sexual deviation, as these have been well documented elsewhere. However, references and suggestions for reading will be given.

As with any other aspect of behaviour, sexual activity has broad limits of what is considered as being normal and acceptable. These limits may vary between cultures, and alter with the course of time.

There are several factors present in a society that can influence the positioning of the limits.

1. Consider (with your group) the significance of the following in the formation of existing attitudes toward sexual behaviour in Great Britain.
religion;
male/female roles;
the mass media;
modern contraceptive techniques;
age.

2. Define what is meant by the term sexual deviation.

ADOLESCENCE

Sexual problems occurring in adolescence differ from other age groups in that they occur in persons whose personalities are not yet fixed, or whose patterns of sexual gratification are rarely completely established.

Additionally, puberty is often late in arriving or seems to take an eternity to achieve its effects!

3. Describe the secondary sexual characteristics associated with puberty:

a. female;
b. male.

Concern over physical development is common in adolescence. Whilst one girl may hunch her shoulders to camouflage her developing breasts; another may look anxiously in the mirror for signs that hers are appearing. For boys, fears usually relate to size of penis and whether they will be big enough to satisfy their partner. Less commonly, they fear they are too big and will hurt their prospective partners.

Sex education is undertaken routinely now in many schools and should ideally take place before the onset of puberty. Despite this, many children seem to enter adolescence poorly informed about sexual behaviour and ignorant about the physical development of their bodies.

4. A female patient on your ward, aged 16, comes to you, confides that she has never had a 'period', and asks if this is normal.

Describe the advice you would give this girl.

Although ignorance with regard both to sexual development and behaviour may be common in adolescence, to be able to readily admit to a need for help is very rare. Peer group status is vitally important during this period and, for males particularly, much bragging takes place concerning recent sexual conquests, both real and imagined. Quite obviously secret fears and feelings of inadequacy may be held but cannot be expressed. If the nurse can anticipate the possible existence of these fears, without them having to be expressed, effective counselling and reassurance can be given in a non-personalised way.

As sexual feelings develop during adolescence, the strength and direction of these is often a cause of great distress for the individual. Adolescence is a time when the individual has a great need to be able to express sexual feelings towards the opposite sex, yet, paradoxically, it is a time when the individual finds it most difficult. Lacking in confidence, feeling awkward and clumsy, and being over-concerned with physical appearance, sexual feelings can often only be expressed as a joke, or in private forms of gratification.

It has been estimated by various reports that masturbation is almost universal amongst boys by the age of 15 or 16. It is less common amongst girls; approximately 25 per cent are said to have masturbated by this age, although this percentage is likely to increase with age groups to a maximum of about 60 per cent in adulthood.

Many claims have been made, both for the physical and psychological benefits of masturbation, and, similarly, for its adverse effects.

5. Consider your own attitude to masturbation. To what extent will your attitude influence any counselling you might give to an adolescent seeking advice on the subject?

If adolescents are experiencing difficulty in adjusting to the opposite sex, it may be easier for them to form sexual relationships with friends of their own sex. Many do during this period, although the relationship does not necessarily include physical contact. Girls particularly may form 'crushes' which may or may not proceed to include physical sexual activity. Boys too may find it easier to indulge in fairly superficial sexual activities with other boys, which may extend to joint masturbation or to masturbating each other. This does not mean that they are likely to be homosexual when they are adult, merely that a homosexual adjustment is easier at that stage of development. In most cases, as confidence with the opposite sex develops, so these early homosexual experiences are forgotten.

Adolescence is a period of great change, both physically and psychologically. The process of achieving an adult personality can be understandably volatile, and the individual often displays types of behaviour that are merely transient phases. This applies to sexual activity as much as to any other aspect of behaviour. For this reason, deviant sexual behaviour occurring in adolescence may just be a transitional phase, and need not indicate serious sexual maladjustment.

It is useful to be aware of the common types of deviant sexual behaviour, if only to be able to discuss these with a little knowledge if approached for advice by a patient. However, expert advice and treatment is required and the nurse who is relatively unskilled in this field should not attempt to give more than supportive reassurance and redirection to where help can be better given.

6. Describe the following briefly:

sexual asphyxia
exhibitionism
fetishism
incest
transvestism

Adolescence is a time of confusion for many young people. It is a time when existing attitudes, ideas and beliefs, many adopted from their parents, are challenged and other often transient ideas replace them. Similarly behaviour too changes, often quite dramatically, as the individual experiments with new styles of behaviour and works towards a personal adult identity. A well-accepted term to describe the difficulties some young people experience during this phase of development is the identity crisis (Erikson). A less common but associated problem that occurs at this time is that of trans-sexuality, in which the individual appears to suffer from a crisis of gender identity. Often such people have from an early age had doubts and confusion about their sex-typing, e.g. they are physically male but feel female.

7. What do you consider the essential characteristics of masculinity and femininity?

8. To what extent is a sense of gender identity and sex role behaviour genetically determined and to what extent is it due to social conditioning?

YOUNG ADULTHOOD

As adolescence is replaced by adulthood, so relationships have a tendency to become more stable and permanent and of course the majority of people marry at this time. For many, the first serious attempt at a fulfilling sexual relationship takes place. Understandably, many couples experience much anxiety and distress during this period as considerable adjustments have to be made.

9. It can be said that it requires less adjustment to form twenty casual sexual relationships than one permanent, successful one.
Consider with your group the implications in the above statement.

Abortive attempts at sexual intercourse during adolescence, particularly when accompanied by an inexperienced or unfeeling partner, frequently lead to disillusionment and foreboding in adulthood. For many individuals sexual technique is learnt by trial and error, and each error is potentially damaging both for donor and recipient! Frequently coupled with ignorance of the human body and how it responds sexually, this combination of events may well result in sexual disaster for many young couples. Shyness and embarrassment may mean that the problem is hidden and not discussed. This in turn can lead to resentment and rejection, which intensifies the original problem. Eventually, the effects will be felt in other areas of the couple's relationship.

Impotence is obviously difficult to conceal, because of the male role in sexual activity, although the sufferer may resort to strategies to avoid sexual intercourse, e.g. complaining of tiredness or of feeling unwell. In our society sexual potency is a vital male attribute, and most men would consider the impotency an affront to their masculinity.

In this age-group anxiety is likely to be the key to causative factor; each episode of failure leads to an increase in anxiety and further reduces the likelihood of the problems being easily overcome.

10. If a young patient were to confide in you that he suffered from impotency, describe what immediate reassurance you could give him.

The equivalent problem in the female is usually referred to as frigidity, although the term orgasmic insufficiency is often preferred, as the former term suggests a 'coldness' that is usually far from the truth! Because of the nature of the female sexual response, orgasmic insufficiency is obviously easier to conceal. Additionally the feminine attitude to orgasm often differs from the masculine attitude. Many women still regard a regular orgasm as a bonus to their lovemaking, and perhaps are more likely to accept a failure to become aroused.

11. The rigid Victorian sexual role for women is well known and is epitomised by the advice of the day to 'close your eyes and think of England' during intercourse.

To what extent do you think that attitude exists today?

Occasionally for some couples intercourse may be impossible because the man's attempts to penetrate his partner's vagina cause painful vaginal muscular spasms (vaginismus).

Frequently becoming parents exerts quite an influence on the couple's sexual relationship. For the new mother there is the physical and psychological recovery to be made, and for both parents some role adjustment is necessary. Many women feel fat and ugly during pregnancy and lose interest in lovemaking. This loss of interest may be aggravated by a fear of injuring the unborn child if intercourse were to be attempted. This fear is quite unfounded, provided the husband is reasonably gentle. Alternative, more comfortable positions for lovemaking can be adopted during pregnancy, and new ways of meeting each other's sexual needs can be experimented with. Often loss of interest continues after the birth and may well cause tension in the relationship if it persists. Patience is a key factor, and provided the husband can be so, and can also be understanding and supportive, a full sexual relationship will be resumed in most cases.

A similar loss of interest in lovemaking can occur in an individual following gynaecological operations such as hysterectomy or tubal ligation. A common fear not readily expressed is that their partners may not find them as sexually attractive as they were. This fear has much in common with the frequent emotional reaction to the menopause (discussed later in the unit). It may be that some women unconsciously associate fertility with sexual desire and that the loss of the former affects the latter. A similar reaction has been reported in men following a vagotomy operation. It should be stressed that the sexual response is not dependent on fertility in any way. Anxieties relating to their future sexual attractiveness are understandably also experienced by many women undergoing mastectomy operations. Despite modern prosthesis and silicone implants they worry that their husbands will find them repugnant. Nurses have an important role in reassuring, supporting and counselling patients who are undergoing such surgery. Often they are reluctant to discuss their anxieties and only indicate their concern in oblique ways such as by making jokes.

12. With reference to patients you have nursed, discuss how the nursing team were able to provide some measure of reassurance.

It is worth pointing out that a loss of interest in lovemaking is understandable in either partner when the basic relationship between them is unhappy or disturbed. This applies to any age group and the sexual problem between them is a symptom of the underlying disturbance.

A problem that occurs almost exclusively in adolescence and young adulthood is that of premature ejaculation. In this the individual ejaculates either prior to penetrating the vagina or almost immediately it is achieved. Although this can be a distressing condition the treatment based on desensitisation, referred to at the end of the unit, is very often successful.

Nurses may be approached by the patient for advice on the quality and frequency of lovemaking. It is important to reassure the patient that there is no rule for either, other than that which satisfies both partners by agreement. Provided both are happy with the nature and frequency of the sexual relationship, then for that couple that is normal. Problems only exist when one or other of the partners feels dissatisifed.

Homosexuality occurring in young adulthood is likely to be a more permanent state than in adolescence, although it may be a compensatory reaction to previous unsuccessful attempts at heterosexual relationships.

13. Discuss the relevance of the following factors in the causation of homosexuality:
hereditary hormonal psychological.

It should be noted that many adult homosexual people are content with their sexual relationships and do not require treatment. Any unhappiness or distress they express is often not a direct result of their sexual status, but of society's often rejecting and prejudicial attitude towards them. This in turn may cause fear, isolation and loneliness.

14. Homosexuality often evokes a fierce over-reaction from heterosexual people. Why might this be so?

MIDDLE AGE

This is often a time of self-evaluation, and unfortunately of disillusionment in many individuals. The aspirations and ambitions of early adulthood may not have been attained. Life may have taken on rather a humdrum tone and many couples may have settled into a reasonably comfortable yet monotonous routine. For such couples it is likely that their sexual relationship has taken on a similar pattern. As the middle years are reached, it is not uncommon for both men and women to experience fears about their sexual prowess, physical appearance and their ability to attract the opposite sex. Such fears may well stem from a fear of growing old, and can motivate behaviour that is inconsistent with a person's previous life style.

15. Describe the type of behaviour changes that might take place.

It has been argued that middle age is more a state of mind than an actual age-range. Interest in the sexual side of a relationship will usually lessen as people grow older. As was mentioned earlier, as long as neither of the partners resents this loss of interest then there will not be a problem. However, if resentment is present then it may cause tension and conflict within the relationship and perhaps end with the dissatisfied partner forming other sexual relationships. Such a loss of interest may be characterised simply by avoidance, or refusal to take part in sexual activity; or it may be an inability to become sexually aroused.

16. Discuss the relevance of the following factors in causing a loss of sexual interest in middle age:
psychogenic psychiatric organic.

17. Patients receiving psychiatric treatment sometimes complain that the drugs they are prescribed seem to be affecting their sexual performance, e.g. failure to achieve and sustain an erection.
Identify the drugs that have side-effects of this nature.

As with childbirth, for many the menopause can result in a change in attitude toward sexual activity. It is not unusual for patients to state that a declining interest in such activity was noticed to coincide with the menopause commencing. Whether this is a result of some hormonal change in the body is debatable. Some women have said that they felt less feminine, and less desirable, when they have become infertile. Ironically, with the fear of pregnancy removed, in many ways this is a time when the sexual aspects of a relationship should become more enjoyable.

18. Comment on the possibility of the existence of a male menopause.

The majority of people in middle age are married or have a permanent relationship with someone. However, for the single person, opportunities for sexual fulfilment are very limited. The typical round of public houses, cinema, or possibly club activities are not likely to provide as many opportunities for acceptable sex as they might for the younger person. Consequently, the single people may be forced to turn to alternative ways of gaining sexual gratification.

19. Discuss the advantages and disadvantages of the following alternatives:
the prostitute;
pornographic books and sex shows;
sublimation.

Unfortunately, for some, alternative sexual fulfilment is not possible or acceptable to them.

20. What effect might the following have on their attitude to sexual behaviour:

denial reaction-formation.

OLD AGE

It is unusual to associate this period of life with problems relating to sexual activity. This probably reflects to a certain extent society's devaluating attitude to the elderly. Certainly many younger people do not consider sexual activity to be important later in life. Probably this is often true, but it is a dangerous generalisation to assume that it applies to all, and may make the minority reluctant to admit to sexual problems.

Every encouragement should be given to those elderly people who wish to continue their sexual relationship. Occasionally, elderly couples may complain that physical frailty or disease inhibits, or even precludes, sexual intercourse. In these situations there is little the nurse can offer, except reassurance and encouragement.

21. Very occasionally, impotence may be a symptom of physical disease. Identify these conditions.

It may happen with some elderly men that disinhibition occurs, possibly as a result of early senile or arteriosclerotic dementia, or simply as an expression of previously suppressed sexual urges. (Refer to the unit on 'nursing the confused patient'.)

Exhibitionism often occurs and occasionally sexual assaults, particularly on children, may take place. This is obviously very distressing for all concerned, particularly as it is usually people of previous good character who are concerned.

On a general note, whenever nurses are approached by patients for help on sexual matters they should never laugh or express disgust. It is not a nurse's duty to moralise or to impose his/her standards of behaviour on others. Patients should be informed of the consequences of being apprehended if their sexual behaviour is illegal, and nurses have a wider duty to society when a patient's sexual behaviour includes unwilling or underage partners. The nurse's main role is to act as a counsellor, giving support and reassurance, and as an educator; also to know when the problem is beyond her individual skills and that further expert guidance is required.

22. Describe your course of action if a patient confided in you that he/she had committed several serious sex crimes.

Problems relating to normal sexual activity may be a feature of some mental illness; however, sexual deviation and sexual crimes are not generally regarded in the same way. They may occur as a *result* of mental illness either because the illness causes a loss of control or inhibition, or because the nature of the illness prevents normal sexual relationships being formed.

23. Using your knowledge of the nature of mental illness, consider which sexual problems/deviations/crimes, might be associated with the following:

depression
psychopathy
hypomania
schizophrenia
alcoholism
hysteria

24. In your opinion, why are sex crimes and sexual deviation more commonly associated with men rather than women?

In addition to mental illness, living in an institution for any length of time may obviously influence an individual's sexual behaviour. Wards are still often single-sex and privacy is at a minimum. Consequently opportunities allowing patients to develop sexual relationships with each other are frequently denied them. Nevertheless sexual liaisons of varying types still manage to flourish in the typical hospital milieu.

25. Discuss with your group what you consider the nursing team's attitude should be towards the following:

a heterosexual relationship between consenting adults.
on a short-stay unit
on a long-stay unit.

A homosexual relationship between consenting adults:
on a short-stay unit
on a long-stay unit.

TREATMENT

Until relatively recently there was very little treatment available for those suffering from sexual disorders. The medical profession could offer some relief to the small percentage of patients whose disorders had an organic basis. The psychiatrist might be involved with those whose psychiatric history included sexual deviation and sexual crime. However, no branch of the medical profession, or any other para-medical profession, has fully accepted the responsibility for the care and treatment of psychosexual disorders. What has often tended to happen is that it has become a shared responsibility between doctors, nurses, psychologists, social workers and other voluntary workers. Although advice and guidance may be given by individuals still, e.g. by general practitioners, the local priest or by community workers, the multidisciplinary team approach is the one that operates from most clinics for psychosexual disorders. Membership of such a team is another example of the extending role of the nurse, but obviously specialist post-basic training is required. For most nurses working in the hospital or community setting, without the specialist training, their role will not extend beyond explanation and education. Such a role should not be belittled, however, as much anxiety can be dispelled by a simple explanation of the facts of sexual activity, particularly with regard to masturbation and the frequency of intercourse. Another area where the nurse can offer advice, with a little necessary research first, is with regard to birth control. Obviously the nurse must always be alert to the patient who needs specialist help in any of these areas, and should be aware of the criteria for referral.

Prior to treatment commencing, any organic causes must be excluded by a thorough physical examination by the doctor. In addition a comprehensive personal and family history is usually required, including religious and social attitudes of the patient and details of sexual development.

26. The more traditional forms of treatment usually involve the following areas. Comment on each one briefly:

suggestion;
relaxation;
manipulation of environment;
psycho-analysis;
conditioning (including aversion therapy);
drugs.

The work of Masters and Johnson's in the treatment of sexual problems has become well known in recent years, and their basic principles have been adopted, at least in part, by many treatment teams. An important aspect of the Masters and Johnson programme is to encourage communication between sexual partners because a basic principle is that *couples* must be treated, and not individuals. In addition, existing sexual attitudes should be identified and modified when relevant to therapy.

Such therapy is usually based on a programme of sensate focus which involves dividing lovemaking into stages and then developing each stage consecutively, in an attempt to reach a predetermined behavioural goal. Sexual intercourse is usually banned at first, and this often gives the couple a great sense of relief. Authoritative direction for sexual behaviour is introduced, and special techniques are taught to the couple.

27. Below are given four examples of special technique. Explain each one briefly:

Diversion (an extension of sensate focus principles).
For erectile impotence and orgasmic insufficiency.

Conditioning (the squeeze techniques).
For premature ejaculation.

De-conditioning (using graded dilators).
For vaginismus.

Unblocking (superstimulation).
For ejaculatory incompetence.

A further Masters and Johnson principle is that therapy is carried out by two therapists, a male and a female (co-therapy). A commitment is sought from the couple to their full co-operation with treatment, and a contract may be drawn up jointly between the co-therapists and the couple, (often referred to as 'conjoint therapy'). Nurses with the relevant training and experience may well become members of such a co-therapy team. Prior to that happening the nurse must obviously have made the adjustment to working in a multi-disciplinary team, as demarcations of authority between therapists do not apply. Additionally they must be prepared to have their own attitudes to sexual behaviour examined closely before they are allowed to treat others.

PROBLEMS RELATING TO SEXUAL ACTIVITY

Self-Evaluation test

Choose the best answer from the alternatives given in each question.

1. The term exhibitionism means:

- **a.** a desire to brag about sexual conquests;
- **b.** a desire to display one's genitals;

c. sexual gratification from watching pornographic films;
d. a desire to parade publicly, dressed in the clothes of the opposite sex.

2. A young man caught stealing female underwear is most likely to be suffering from:

a. voyeurism;
b. homosexuality;
c. kleptomania;
d. fetishism.

3. A key factor in the causation of trans-sexualism is thought to be:

a. faulty gender-role identification;
b. a chromosomal deficiency;
c. an over-protective mother;
d. sibling rivalry.

4. An unreasonably rigid, suppressive attitude to matters relating to sexual activity may well be an example of:

a. displacement;
b. denial;
c. projection;
d. reaction-formation.

5. A loss of desire for lovemaking is common in young mothers in the months following child-birth. This is mainly because of:

a. fatigue following the birth;
b. breast feeding making it difficult;
c. anxiety created by role adjustment;
d. vaginal damage resulting from the birth.

6. Premature ejaculation can usually successfully be treated by a technique based on:

a. conditioning;
b. de-conditioning;
c. diversion;
d. sublimation.

Assertion and reason

Each of the questions in this section consist of an assertion followed by a reason. Assign to each question one of the five categories (a–e) in the key below.

KEY

a. The assertion and reason are both true.
The reason is a correct explanation of the assertion.

b. The assertion and reason are both true.
The reason is *not* a correct explanation of the assertion.

c. The assertion is true but the reason is false.

d. The assertion is false but the reason is true.

e. The assertion and reason are both false.

ASSERTION
1. Most homosexuals display personality traits of the opposite sex.

REASON
Homosexuality can be regarded as a desire to change sex.

ASSERTION
2. Masturbation frequently results in feelings of guilt during adolescence.

REASON
Adolescents are frequently ignorant of the facts regarding masturbation because embarrassment causes the subject to be avoided by parents.

ASSERTION
3. Patients with sexual problems should be counselled by nurses who are tolerant of such problems.

REASON
It is important that counsellors are not emotionally involved when giving guidance to patients.

ASSERTION
4. Generally it is advisable to assign a rate of intercourse to couples who are having sexual difficulties.

REASON

Norms of lovemaking can only be assessed in individual couples and not generalised.

ASSERTION

5. A loss of personal drive may occur during middle age, and this often extends to sexual activity.

REASON

Middle-aged couples may unconsciously adjust their life-style to avoid sexual contact and confrontation when a loss of interest in lovemaking occurs.

True/false items

1. Men and women have the same sex hormones in their bodies but the amounts differ. (True; False)
2. Sex hormones have little influence over physical masculine/feminine attributes. (True; False)
3. The size of the erect penis is directly related to sexual adequacy. (True; False)
4. Women have the same amount of sex drive as men. (True; False)
5. The process of puberty is generally constant in most adolescents. (True; False)
6. Sexual problems occurring in adolescence are often transitory. (True; False)
7. Sexual activity is important to peer group status during adolescence. (True; False)
8. Most youngsters enter adolescence today well-informed and properly educated about sexual activity. (True; False)
9. Sexual difficulties are often indicative of deeper relationship problems. (True; False)
10. Failure of communication is thought to be a key causative factor in marital sexual disorders. (True; False)

REFERENCES AND SUGGESTIONS FOR FURTHER READING

Allen, C. (1969), *A Textbook of Psychosexual Disorders*, Oxford University Press.

Bancroft, J. (1976), 'The Masters and Johnson Approach in a N.H.S. Setting', *British Journal of Sexual Medicine*, **1**, no, 8.

Barnes, K. C. (1970), *He and She*, Penguin.
Holdsworth, A. V. (1978). *Sex Problems in Marriage*, 20 July edition of *Nursing Mirror*.
Haslam, M. T. (1978), *Sexual Disorders*, Pitman Medical.
Irwin, E. M. (1977), *Growing Pains*, MacDonald & Evans.
Kaplan, H. S. (1974), *The New Sex Therapy*, Baillière Tindall.
Masters, W. H. and Johnson, W. E. (1966), *Human Sexual Response*, Little Brown.
——, (1976), *Human Sexual Inadequacy*, Granada Publishing Ltd.
Parker, T. (1969), *The Twisting Lane – some Sex Offenders*, Panther.
Pomeroy, W. B. (1968), *Boys and Sex*, Pelican.
——, (1969), *Girls and Sex*, Pelican.
Randell, J. (1977), *Transsexualism and its Management*, 24 March edition of *Nursing Mirror*.
Schofeld, M. (1968), *The Sexual Behaviour of Young People*, Pelican.
Storr, A. (1964), *Sexual Deviation*, Pelican.
Trimmer, E. (1978), *Basic Sexual Medicine*, Heinemann.

Answers

Unit 1 Mental Health

Multiple Choice

1. a
2. c
3. b
4. b
5. d
6. b
7. a
8. d
9. c

Assertion and Reason

1. a
2. c
3. a
4. d
5. b
6. a

True/False Items

1. F
2. T
3. T
4. F
5. F
6. T
7. F
8. T
9. T
10. T

Unit 2 The Nurse–Patient Relationship

Multiple Choice

1. c
2. b
3. c
4. iv
5. c
6. c

Assertion and Reason

1. a
2. d
3. a
4. d
5. e
6. a
7. c
8. a

True/False Items

1. T
2. T
3. T
4. F
5. F
6. T

Unit 3 Nursing the Depressed Patient

Multiple Choice

1. b,d,e,g
2. a,d,e
3. c
4. a,e,f
5. d
6. a
7. c
8. b

Assertion and Reason

1. c
2. d
3. a
4. a
5. c
6. b

7. b
8. e

True/False Items

1. T
2. F
3. F
4. T
5. F
6. T
7. T
8. T

Unit 4 Nursing the Anxious Patient

Multiple Choice

1. d
2. d
3. d
4. c
5. d
6. ii
7. b
8. c
9. c
10. b

Assertion and Reason

1. a
2. b
3. a
4. c
5. a
6. b
7. a
8. d
9. d
10. a

True/False Items

1. F
2. F
3. T
4. F
5. T
6. T

7. T
8. T
9. F
10. F

Unit 5 The Problem of Aggression

Multiple Choice

1. b
2. d
3. a
4. b
5. c
6. a
7. d

Assertion and Reason

1. c
2. a
3. b
4. a
5. b
6. a
7. a
8. e

True/False Items

1. T
2. T
3. F
4. T
5. F
6. T
7. T
8. F
9. F
10. T

Unit 6 Nursing the Confused Patient

Multiple Choice

1. b,c,f
2. e,c
3. iv
4. b
5. d
6. d,e

7. d
8. c
9. iv
10. a,c,d

Assertion and Reason

1. c
2. c
3. e
4. a
5. a
6. a
7. a
8. b
9. d
10. a
11. b

True/False Items

1. T
2. T
3. F
4. T
5. F
6. T
7. T
8. F
9. T
10. T
11. T

Unit 7 Nursing Patients Dependent on Drugs and Alcohol

Multiple Choice

1. d
2. b
3. c
4. a
5. iv
6. c
7. a
8. b

Assertion and Reason

1. b
2. e

3. b
4. d
5. a
6. a

True/False Items

1. F
2. T
3. T
4. F
5. T
6. T
7. F
8. T
9. T
10. T

Unit 8 The Care of the Suspicious Patient

Multiple Choice

1. a
2. a
3. c
4. c
5. c
6. iv

Assertion and Reason

1. a
2. c
3. a
4. a
5. d
6. a
7. e

True/False Items

1. T
2. T
3. F
4. T
5. T
6. F

Unit 9 Nursing the Withdrawn Patient

Multiple Choice

1. c
2. b,d
3. d
4. c
5. a
6. ii
7. d
8. c,d

Assertion and Reason

1. a
2. e
3. a
4. a
5. a
6. c
7. a
8. d

True/False Items

1. F
2. T
3. T
4. F
5. F
6. T

Unit 10 Problems Relating to Sexual Activity

Multiple Choice

1. a
2. d
3. a
4. d
5. c
6. a

Assertion and Reason

1. e
2. a
3. a
4. b
5. b

True/False Items

1. T
2. F
3. F
4. T
5. F
6. T
7. T
8. F
9. T
10. T

Index